Dr. Hale's Home Remedy & Recipe Book

A DOCTOR'S HANDWRITTEN HANDBOOK
WRITTEN BETWEEN 1844 AND 1863

RESTORED BY
DOUGLAS B. SHARP

EABooks Publishing
Your Partner In Publishing

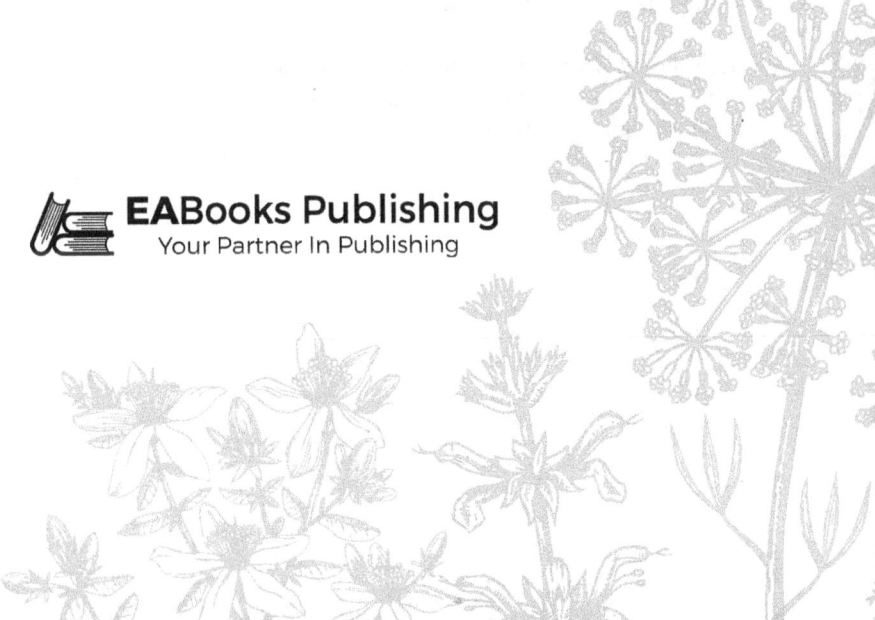

Dr. Hale's Home Remedy and Recipe Book, A Doctor's Handwritten Handbook, Written Between 1844 and 1863
By Dr. Wallace A. Hale, Restored by Douglas B. Sharp
Copyright © 2022

Special acknowledgements to Dr. Wallace A. Hale, Jerome H. Hale, Lucy M. Hale, Fannie E. Hale and Benjamin F. Hale for their contributions to the original book.

All rights reserved. No part of this book may be used or reproduced by any means—graphic, electronic, or mechanical—including photocopying, recording, taping or by any information storage retrieval system without the written permission of the author except in the case of brief quotations embodied in critical articles and reviews.

ISBN 13: 978-1-953114-86-0
LCCN: 2022918636

Cover Art: iStockphoto.com
Author photo courtesy of Douglas B. Sharp
All other photos from the author's personal album

Published by EA Books Publishing, a division of
Living Parables of Central Florida, Inc. a 501c3
EABooksPublishing.com

TABLE OF CONTENTS

(Note: spelling as original pages)

Introduction by Douglas B. Sharp	15
Transcribing the Handwritten Pages	22
English System of Weights and Measures 1828–1864	23
Poison for Rats Steal not this book, you little cusses…	24
J. H. Hale and Lucy M. Hale's Book Cass County, Michigan	26
This Book belongs to W. A. Hale Ann Arbor, Mich.	28
Mr. Book, If thou art borrowed by a friend… Rent commenced Aug. 17, 1846	30
This Book Belongs to Wallace A. Hale To My Book…	32
Cure for the Canker Vegetable Powder Code at the bottom	34
Wallis Cough Med	36
Compound Zinc Myrrh, Alias No 6 Vegetable Bitters	38
Vegetable Ointment Vegetable Syrup for Dysentary	40
Worm Syrup Dysentary	42
Cough Emulsion Sore Eyes	44

Lees Pill Quick Pill No. 1 Ague Pill Ague Pill (note Arsenic in coded ingredient)	46
Ague (continued) For Cornes Pulmonary Mixture	48
Venerial Alias Clap Spruce Beer	50
Diarhoea Hiera Picra Cough Drops New Vegetable Physic	52
Spruce Beer Itch Ointment Compound Balsam Ginger Beer	54
Gox Medicine Cure for Gravel Good for the Itch Ague Bitters	56
For Bots and Belly Ache in Horses Itch Ointment Medical or Root Beer	58
Rhumatic Liniment Black Salve	60
Best Adhesive Plaster Rx Fever and Ague	62
Ammenagogue For Gonnorhoea or Clap	64
My Emetic	66

Diarrhoea or Bowel Disease Carbonated Beer Ginger Beer	68
Pill Pargantia Ice Cream	70
Ice Cream (continued) Corn Meal Cakes	72
Genuine Whigs Cookies Another Wafers Jumbles	74
Cookies Nut Cake Muffins Number Cake Rusks	76
Measure Cake Little Cake Sponge Cake Plum Cake	78
Crockers Ginger Bread Fruit Cake Puff Paste York Bisket	80
Whip Sillabub Common Loaf Cake Icing for Cake	82

The Real John Bull Pudding Cookies Again Harrison Cake	84
Cream Cake Sunderland Pudding Pound Cake Kings Cake Indelable Ink	86
To Colour Green Pound Cake will keep 1 year Pudding	88
Birds Nest Pudding Ginger Bread Cider Cake	90
Bread To Cure Warts Soft Gingerbread Cookies French Loaf	92
Imitation Oysters To Clean Gloves Good Custard	94
To Clean Bed Ticks To make a soiled coat look as good as new	96
To Extract Greace Spots	98
To make Sweet Cider To make Japan Liquid Blacking	100
Mead To make Cream Nectar	102

To make good vinegar Housels Washing Solution Patented July 7, 1848	104
Medicated Indian Oil	106
Shure cure for stifle in horses	108
To take Mildew out of linen To set fast colours in calico and other goods To perfume clothes and prevent moths Cheap paint To cure hams	110
Water Proof for Leather Valuable Eye water Chil Blains To banish mosquitoes	112
How to cut an acquaintance Brandy Red Adhesive Plaster Cough Med	114
Eye Matter For the Croup Staining guns	116
For the Croup by B. F. Hale Dropsy by B. F. Hale Gum Salve	118
Mathers Stomach Bitters or Cordial My Bathing drops	120
Phloridzin To remove pimpels from the face	122
Dr. Hales best linement Eye Matter	124

Tooth Ache For ringworm My best linement For neuralgia	126
Cancer plaster	128
For pain in stomach, bowels, diarrhea, cholera morbus, spasm, colic and for external use with nervous pains Diptheria Rheumatic Liniament	130
Itch Ointment Cement for Uniting My Cupping Glasses Fit Drops for Epilepsy Infalible Healing Salve	132
Warms Blue Cohush, its properties and uses Lucy's Ague Cough Balsam	134
Nerve and Bone Linneament Cough Powders	136
Worm Lozenges For the Cea Ginger	138
Rheumatic Linneament	140
Cholera Med Grand Ague Med Cornes	142
Black Salve Cologn Matter	144
Gran Salve Good Sweet-tinct Rheubarb Lucys last cough med	146

Hydrophobia Diarrhoea Annother	148
Allerative for C. Harts little child Dr. Hale's Stomach bitters or cordial	150
Dr. Hales Sameritan Lineament	152
Anothers very excellent med for pain in bowels Discutient Ointment	154
Spasmodic Atackts Syrup for the lungs	156
Dysmenorrhea or painful menstruation	158
Dr. Hale's best and last liver pills Thunder and Lightening Cough Medicine B. F. Hale	160
Dysenteric Med Cordials Ague Pills, my last	162
White Liquid Physic Powerful Nervine Gonerrhoea Infection	164
Gonorrhoea Bleeding of the lungs Fever sores	166
Stomach Cordial Eruption on the face	168
Liver Powders by B. F. Hale Liver Drops	170
Simple Cerate Rheumatic Tinct	172

Rheumatism Linneament for sprains, bruises, strains, or Rheumatism Vermafuge	174
Gonorrhoea	176
For Tape Worm Plaster for Tape Worms Excellent Cologne Watter Carminative or Infant Cordial	178
Worms—a good vermifuge Cough Med	180
Lip Salve For Cough Eye Wash To remove films Sticking salve	182
Dr. Hale's Cholera Syrup Black Linneament	184
Rx Pomade for restoring the hair Nervine and Carminative Balsam	186
Conklin's Salve Lords Salve Cholera drops	188
Pain Killer For Goitre, swelled neck, Serofulous Cancers, Tumors	190
Colyrium or Eye Matter Diarrhoea Colera morbus	192

Salt–Rhumi Ointment Pills for Dropsy Emmenagogue Tinct	194
Spice Bitters Cutaneuous Cancers—to be tried for outer ringworm, warts, moles cornes Comp tinct Camphor	196
Pery Davises Pain Killer Kitridge Nerve Ointment Bone Linneament	198
Scrofula Pill Com tinct Camphor Rheumatic Drops	200
Chilblains Dr. Allens Cholera Syrup	202
Comp Ointment Ptramonium	204
For Cough Nerve and Bone Linneament	206
Dyspeptic Powders Cutaneous Ointment Spermacite Cough balsam	208
Lavendar Matter Palpitation	210
Rx Bitters Ointment for the Eye Cough Drops	212
Cough Drops Cough Powders	214

For Cholera Plaster Linneament for people	216
Sure Cure for Hydrophobia Cornes For Piles	218
For one qt of Hellenium Balsam For Neuralgia	220
Cholera Med Heitridge Nerve Ointment To prepare soap	222
Salve Rheumatism Tinct	224
Heitridge's Ointment For dysentery, dyarrehoea	226
Cement for cisterns Godfrey's Cordial Wallace's Cough Medicine	228
Quinz Cologne Remedy called Cureall	230
Ointment for Tinea Capitis or Scale Head Blistering Plaster Linneament Sacrid	232
Stramonium Ointment Rx for Staining gun barrels	234
To case harden by S. A. J. Hale Antiphlogistic or Cooling Plaster Indian Salve	236

For Ague and Fever Composition Improved Alternative	238
Liver Syrup	240
Horse and Man Linneament Diptheria	242
Last Alternative Another Strengthening Plaster	244
Last Alternative	246
Chronic Rheumatism Suderific Drops	248
Injection for Gonorrhoea Vegitable Salve	250
Chry Pectoral Sulphate	252
Rx for making vegitable oil to burn in lamps superior to oil or gass Syrup Sassaprilla for the blood, Syphilis, Scrofula, and all Impurities of the circulating fluid	254
To Produce Salination Gonorrhoea	256
For Lungs and Liver	258
Diarrhoea	260
Hydro Alcoholic Ext Blue Cohush	262
Vegitable Drops	264
Corn Tinc Lobelia Syrup of Wild Cherry	266
Conf Syrup of Rheubarb Neutralizing Cordial	268
Indian Linneament	270

Elderberry Wine Good Black Ink	272
Obviating Syrup Chill Fever & Ague	274
For another Neuralgia & pain in the head	276
Itch Ointment Plaster Fever Sore	278
Clap or Gonorrhoea	280
Phymosis Paraphymosis Paint thinner	282
Cholic Stomach Pills Annother Strenghtening plaster Plaster for old sores Mother's relief For the blood	284
Catarrh Snuff Lucys Cold Bitters Adhesive Plaster	286
For captive habits Pill Coating	288
Index to this book (Dr. Hale using original pages)	290–311
Back pages	312–313
Index of Ingredients	314–332
Index of Diseases	333
Food, Other Recipes, Miscellaneous	339

Introduction by Douglas B. Sharp

This unique handwritten book was found in a trunk in my grandmother's attic about in the 1980's along with a collection of books dating from 1859-1915. We often wondered about its origin and the family who wrote it.

My grandmother was Thelma M. Sharp, and we presumed that these books came from the house in Lewiston, Michigan she inherited from her uncle Elmer Thompson. We used this house as a vacation home in the 1960's. The Lewiston house was built by a lumber-man, Otis Kneeland, in 1890 and was one of only three houses that survived the fires that burned down this town during the lumber days. That house was next door to the David Kneeland house, where the Lewiston Historical Society now has a museum. David Kneeland was the manager of the Salling, Hanson & Company in Lewiston and Grayling, and later owned the Kneeland-Bigelow Lumber Company.

One day a few years ago I came upon a reference to a 1913 book about the history of Calhoun County that matched the names in this book. The reference was about Walter F. Hale, brother to the principal author of this book Wallace A. Hale. Here is what it reads:

WALTER F. HALE: By thirty or more years of successful activity as an agriculturist Walter F, Hale has earned a place on the roster of Calhoun county's representative citizens and deserves mention among those who have been valued factors in the upbuilding of Clarence township. Himself a native son of Michigan, he is a scion of two of this state's pioneer settlers and has other ancestral inheritance of more than usual interest. The Hales were a prominent colonial family of the old Massachusetts commonwealth and Walter F. Hale as the distinction of being the grandson of Nathaniel Wallace, an aide to General Washington during the Revolution.

Born in Cass county, Michigan, October 16, 1844, Walter F. Hale is a son of Jerome H. and Lucy (Wallace) Hale, pioneers of Michigan who were residents of the state many years. The father was born in Massachusetts in 1824 and when a boy came to Michigan with his parent in 1836, the family spending their first winter in Detroit but later re-moving to Niles. After he had taken up independent responsibilities, he became a merchant at Wauconda, Illinois, where he remained a number of years , or until 1857, when failing in business, he returned to Michigan, which state thereafter remained his home. After his return here he followed carpentering until his death and was fairly successful. In politics he was a Republican and took an active and leading part in the local affairs of his party. While a resident of Wauconda, Illinois, he served as postmaster six years and was a candidate for treasurer but was defeated on account of his strong dislike of slavery. He was a son of Dr. Benjamin F. Hale who, as previously mentioned, came to Michigan in 1836. He was a physician of skill and spent the remainder of his life in this state as an active practitioner at Ann Arbor and Ypsilanti, passing away in 1869. Lucy (Wallace) Hale, the mother of our subject, was born in New York in 1826 and was the daughter of Nathaniel Wallace, the Revolutionary patriot referred to above who served seven years in the struggle for national independence and was an aide to General Washington. He was a native of New York and was a wealthy silk merchant. Mrs. Hale drew a pension for his war service. She was a regular attendant of the Presbyterian church.

Walter F. Hale is one of two sons that came to his parents, the other being Wallace Hale, now deceased. He received good educational advantages, his preliminary studies in the common schools of Wauconda, Illinois, having been supplemented by a period of study in the academy at Wauconda and by two years' work in the University of Michigan, Ann Arbor. He began business activity as a photographer and followed that line of endeavor three years. At the end of that period, he took up farming, on the shares until his marriage in 1874, and after that independently on his present homestead of fifty-six acres in Clarence township, where his attention has since been given to general farming and to peach raising, having a fine large orchard of this fruit on his place. In political views and affiliations, he is a Republican and in an official way has served as constable, township clerk, highway commissioner and as township supervisor in 1902 and 1903. Mrs. Hale was Miss Jennie Bell prior to her marriage, a daughter of Oliver S. Bell and Reliance M. (Dixon) Bell, who were highly respected pioneer residents of Clarence township. Mr. Bell was born in New York in 1816 and came to Calhoun county, Michigan, in 1836, locating on an eighty-acre farm in Clarence township which afterward remained his residence until his death in 1874. His wife, who also was a native of New York, was born in 1823 and died in 1904, at the advanced age of eighty-one years. Andrew Bell, the grandfather of Mrs. Hale, was a soldier in the war of 1812. The education of Mrs. Hale included a term at Albion College. Three children have blessed the union of Mr. and Mrs. Hale, namely: Frederick, who married Eva Graham and who manages the home place; Nellie, who married Charles Sabin and Maude, the wife of Edward Van Sickle, who resides in Clarence township, and who was a soldier in the Spanish-American war. They also have six interesting grandchildren: Orvil O. Hale; Walter C. and Aaron O., the sons of Mr. and Mrs. Sabin; and Frederick, Ethel and Edwin, the children of Mr. and Mrs. Van Sickle.

The discovery of this reference caused me to wonder if there were any descendants of this family still in Michigan. I found Orvil O. Hale in a 1940 census with two children named Jerome and Truman. Then, I found Truman Hale in Farwell, Michigan with an Internet search and he had a telephone number, so I called him up. I began to describe to him what I had found, and he verified that his father was Orvil, his grandfather was Frederick and great-grandfather was Walter. I sent him a copy of this book that I had scanned onto a DVD.

Then Truman referred me to his sister Lois Hale Reid, who is the family historian, and she said that Wallace was a physician in Ashley, Michigan, and that years ago she had his doctor's bag with all the tools. But one day it disappeared. She also has another book like this one, and it is likely the "large book" referred to on pages 16 and 45 in this book. Her brother Jerome had died as a child. I also am in contact with Jeff Hale, Truman's son, and Angie Reid-Garcia,

Lois' daughter. Jeff lives in the Clarence township area referenced in this book.

Since I have been volunteering as a docent at the Michigan History Center in Lansing, I made the decision to donate the original copy of this book to the State of Michigan Archives, where you can view it upon special request. Along with this, I donated a collection of photograph post cards by Elmer Thompson and a ledger from the ghost town of Summitville in Lake County with poetry, drawings, and entries from 1839–1872.

Now the question still remains how this document ended up with Elmer Thompson's belongings, then with my grandmother and finally given by her to me. Elmer owned several resort properties in northern Michigan according to the stories my father told me, he was a bit of a rascal. The big house in Kneeland Street in Lewiston was rented out to hunters and fisherman.

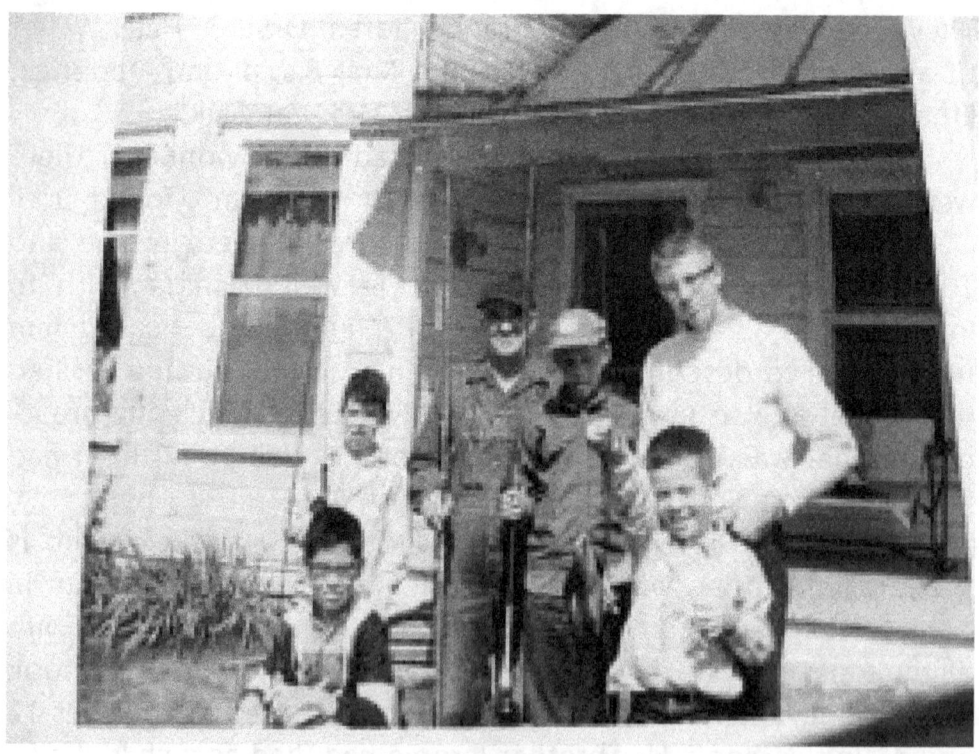

The Big House at Lewiston where this book was found

He owned a cabin on East Twin Lake, and since that lake wasn't that good for fishing, he would catch a mess of fish at other nearby lakes and have it in a cage by the dock so that people would rent his cabin for fishing. Once he was skinning a deer out of season in his front yard, and the game warden lived across the street. Someone passing by asked him if he was afraid of being caught. "Naah", he exclaimed. "He's out in the woods looking for violators."

Elmer also had built a cabin out in the woods near McCormick Lake and dammed up a stream for a waterwheel to power his cabin with electricity. His photo album (also in the archives) also shows several camps he owned on Loon Lake and Higgins Lake.

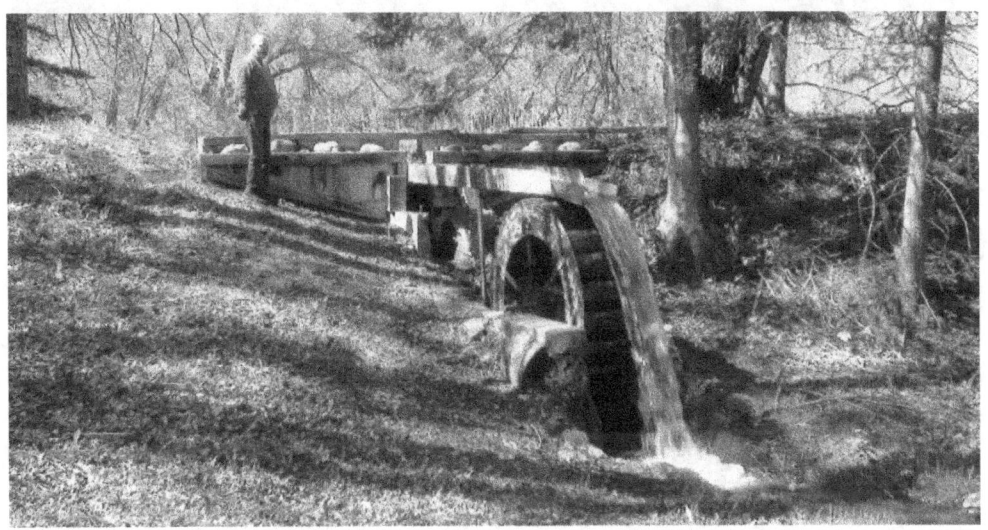

Elmer's Waterwheel at Thompson Pond near Lewiston

But he also had a farm in Clarence township near Albion in Calhoun county, and that would put him in the neighborhood of the Hale farm. My speculation is that, despite all of the warnings in the beginning of the book not to "steal this book, you little cusses" and to return this book if borrowed, Elmer somehow borrowed this book, probably from either Frederick, Orvil, or Wallace himself, and never returned it.

This book is fascinating to read and depicts the kind of life a doctor would have between 1846 to 1863. On page 1 at the bottom,

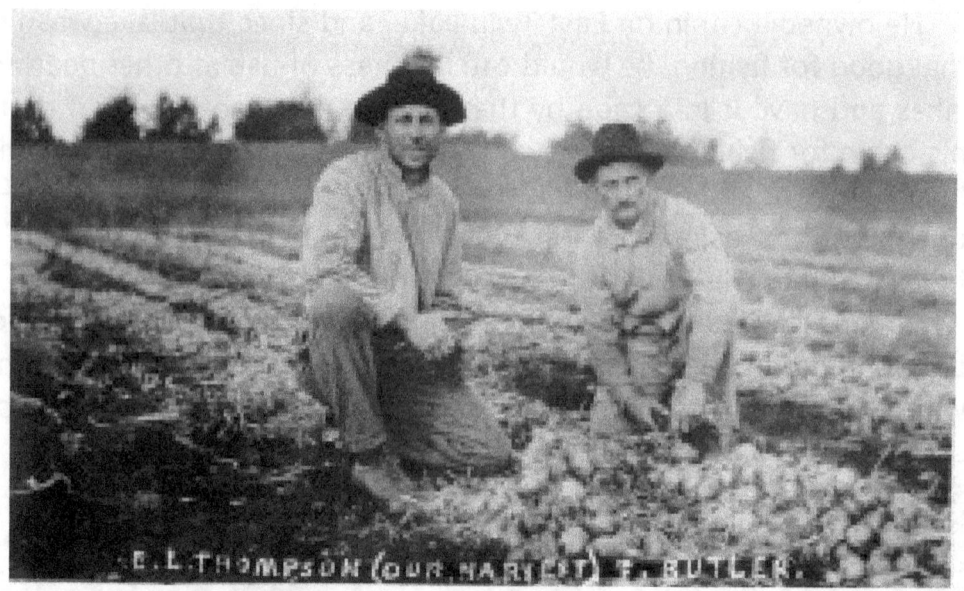

there is an alphabetic code that the writer invented. Elsewhere in the book, such as the pill for Ague on page 7, he writes certain ingredients in that code. In this case, he is putting arsenic in this pill. The Victorian script is sometimes a little hard to read, and the writer is inconsistent in his spelling. But this book would have captured the essence of the life of this doctor, and it would have been a very valuable possession.

Some of the prescriptions may not have worked very well, as they are crossed off. A majority of them come from his grandfather Benjamin F. Hale and there are also entries from Jerome, Lucy, and Fannie. The final page shows the plan of J. H. Hale's house in Wauconda, Illinois.

Some of the remedies and recipes may still be in use today, and they might be worthwhile to try, such as "Bird's Nest Pudding" on page 29. The recipes for Mead on page 35 and Ice Cream on page 19-20 are fascinating, especially the part about sawing a barrel in two to build the ice cream freezer apparatus.

I am hoping that restoring this book, reprinting it, and making it available for other people to read will honor the history of the Hale family and open up more understanding of what life was like in Michigan's past. If, indeed, my great-great uncle borrowed this book from the Hale family 100 years ago and never returned it, now it has completed its circuit, and been restored, finally to be reproduced again to tell the life story of a pioneer doctor in Michigan.

Transcribing the Handwritten Pages

It was an extreme challenge to read these handwritten pages and transcribe them so that they would be readable. I have done this with facing pages so you can see the original as well as the typeset version. Ingredients were looked up, misspellings were corrected, and references were made where appropriate.

By no means do I recommend duplicating these recipes and using them as cures, especially the ones that use mercury, lead, rhodium, arsenic, and other poisons. This compilation is to give a picture of historical medicinal practices. It is interesting to find cures here that are still used today. But as you can see, some of these were crossed off . . . oops . . . must not have worked. . . .

However, some of the breads, puddings, cakes, and drinks might be interesting to try, and the historic ice cream recipe that talks about making the freezing apparatus is fascinating.

The system of weights and measures is the traditional English apothecary system used from 1828 to 1864. What follows is a table of conversion of these to what is more commonly used today.

English System of Weights and Measures
1828-1864

Weight Abbr.	Pound ℔	Ounce ℥, oz	Drachm ʒ	Scruple ℈	Grain gr
	1 ℔	12 ℥	96 ʒ	288 ℈	5,760 gr
		1 ℥	8 ʒ	24 ℈	480 gr
			1 ʒ	3 ℈	60 gr
				1 ℈	20 gr
Metric Equivalent	373 g	31.1 g	3.89 g	1.296 g	64.8 mg
Post 1864	1 lb	16 oz			7000 gr
Metric Equivalent	455 g	28.3 g			64.8 g

Quantities are expressed in Roman numerals and often used Latin syntax. For example, four ounces would be expressed as ℥iv, three drachms as ʒiij, with the j preventing tampering with or misinterpreting the number after it is written. ½ drachm would be expressed as ʒss, with the ss representing "semis." In this book, the handwritten drachm symbol is not that much different from the ounce symbol so there are likely mistakes in my interpretation.

Other weights and measures:

1 gill = ½ cup

do = dozen?

Where an ingredient is first used, I will make a note about it if it isn't commonly known. I will also refer back to that page when appropriate. Use the ingredient index in back to find the first reference.

powd Assafaetida ½ gr
oil if Anniseed one drachm
essential oil of Lavender one scruple
do oil Rhodium 3 drachms
mix this compound and spread
in or the bait in trap
poison for Rats

Steal not this book
You little curses
For if you do you will
Hear of curses

(Inside cover)

Powder Asafetida ¼ gr
Oil of Anise seed one drachm
Essential oil of Lavender one scruple
Do Oil Rhodium 3 drachms
Mix this compound and spread it on the bait in trap
Poison for Rats

Steal not this book
You little cusses
For if you do you will
Hear of fusses

P. H. Hales &
Lucy M. Hales Book

Cass County
                Michigan

This Book is full of
Usefull Knowledge
to the Oner P. H. H.
Recpt Book
        Hands off — Leave Book

When this book of any choice to
Remember that it belong to one
            P H Hal

J. H. Hales &
Lucy M. Hale's Book
Cass County, Michigan

This book is full of Useful Knowledge to the Owner
J.H.H. Recipe[1] Book
Hands off Book
When this book you choose to see
Remember that it belongs to me
W. A. Hale

---

1 Note recipe was spelled "receipt" back then.

This Book belongs
To
W A Hale
Ann Arbor
Mich

This Book contains
361 Receipts
Written by
P. H. Hale
Wallace A Hale
Fannie E Hale and B. F. Hale

This Book belongs
To
W. A. Hale
Ann Arbor, Mich
This book contains
361 Receipts
Written by
J. H. Hale
Wallace A. Hale
Fannie E. Hale and B. F. Hale

My Book

If thou art Borrowed by a friend
rite welcome shall he be to read
to Stranger not to lend but to return to
me
Books are often lent & I
want them returned with their
corners not turned down.
A Word to the wise is
Sufficient
B. F. Hale

Rent Commenced Aug 17 1846
Amount of rent per year $35,00
Philip Weart

Adamsville Aug 17 1845
Between Philip Weart & B. F. Hale

Wallace A. Hale
Geneva Courthouse
Va.

Mr. Book
If thou art borrowed by a friend
Right welcome shall he be to read
To study not to lend but to return to me
Books are often lent & I
Want them returned with their corners not turned down
A word to the wise is sufficient.
J. H. Hale
Rent commenced Aug. 17, 1846
Amount of rent per year $35.00 Philip Weart
Adamsville Aug 17, 1846
Between Philip Weart and B. F. Hale
Wallace A. Hale
Geneva Courthouse, Va.

This Book
Belongs to Doctor A. H. ...

To my book

If thou art borrowed by a friend,
Right welcome shall he be,
To read, to study, not to lend,
But to return to me.

Not that imparted knowledge doth
  Diminish learnings store,
But Books I find if often lent
Return to me no more.

Wallaceville, Dec 24th 1863
Michigan.

Read slowly, pause frequently,
Think seriously,
Keep cleanly, Return duly,
with the corners of the leaves
not turned down.

This Book
Belongs to Wallace A. Hale

To my book
If thou art borrowed by a friend
Right welcome shall he be
To read to study not to lend
But to return to me.
Not that imparted knowledge doth
Diminish learnings store
But if Books I find if often lent
Return to me no more.

Wallaceville, Michigan* Dec. 24th, 1863
Read slowly pause frequently
Think seriously
Keep cleanly Return duly
With the corners of the leaves
Not turned down
*Wallaceville was near present day Garden City, Michigan, incorporated in 1862 and ceased being a post office in 1901.

Universal Rect Book

Cure for the Canker

A Strong tea made of red rospberry laves and drink freely is good. The leaves of Witch hazle Sumac berries bark or leaves or the root of pon billies made into a Strong tea is good in this case

Vegetable Powder

Take one lb of babery bark of the root dried pound fine and Sift through a fine Sive four oz of iner bark of the common hemlock (having Shaved off the ross) Pound fine and Sift do Eight oz of Ginger four oz of Cayenne pepper four oz of witch hazle dried pounded fine and Sift as the others two oz of Cloves pounded and Sifted mix all well togher and they are fit for use

Universal Recipe Book

Cure for the Canker

A Strong tea made of red raspberry leaves and drink freely is good. The leaves of witch hazel, sumac, berries, bark or leaves or the root of pond lilies[1] made into a strong tea is good in this case.

Vegetable Powder

Take one ℔ [pound] of bayberry[2] bark of the root, dried, pound fine and sift through a fine sieve. Four oz of inner bark of the common hemlock (having shaved off the roots). Pound fine and sift, do eight oz of ginger, four oz of cayenne pepper, four oz of witch hazel, dried, pounded fine and sift as the others, two oz of cloves pounded and sifted, mix all well together and they are fit for use.

Note: At the bottom of this page there exists a code where Doctor Hale encrypts certain ingredients in his formulas. Where this exists, I will translate accordingly. However some of these are still difficult to interpret. I will flag the encoded ingredients. If I am unable to identify the ingredient, I will put a question mark after it. If you think my transcription is incorrect, I would appreciate your input!

A B C D E F G H I J K L M N O P Q R S T U V W X Y Z

---

1   Nuphar, an astringent
2   Morella pensylvanica

A good Article for Children

Wallis Cough Med

Blood root one drachm Spikenard root 4 drachms Digitatis 1/2 drachm Comfry root 3 drachms hourhoun 2 drachms boil all in pt of whiskey & a quart of water boil 8 times & pour off. bring it down after Straining to one pt add 4 oz honey boil 3 minutes & Skim when cold ~~add one gr of tartarized antimony disolved in a little warm water~~ to every oz Syrup add one drachm best tincture of lobelia Shake well..... Add to the above 4 oz good raisins & a pt more of water & 2 oz of loaf Sugar & Stick Liquirice 2 drachm

Dose Commence with a small tea Spoonfull and increase the dose untill a little Sickness is got up If hot wither add a little Spirits

A good Article for Children

Wallis Cough Medicine

Bloodroot[3] one drachm[4], spikenard[5] root 4 drachms, digitalis ½ drachm, comfrey[6] root 3 drachms, horehound[7] 2 drachms, boil all in a pint of whiskey and a quart of water. Boil 8 times and pour off. Bring it down after straining to one pint, add 4 ounces of honey, boil 3 minutes and skim when cold. To every oz syrup add one drachm best tincture of lobelia.[8] Shake well, add to the above 4 oz of good raisins and a pint more of water and 2 oz of loaf sugar and stick licorice 2 drachms.

Dose: Commence with a small teaspoonful and increase the dose until a little sickness is got up. If hot weather, add a little spirits.

*a drachm is 1/8 of an ounce or 60 grains.

---

3   a North American plant of the poppy family
4   a drachm is 1/8 of an ounce or 60 grains.
5   Himalayan plant of the valerian family
6   a Eurasian plant of the borage family
7   Used as an expectorant
8   a chiefly tropical or subtropical plant of the bellflower family

X Compound Tinc Myrrh _Alias_ No 6 good for pain in bowels very hot — 3

Alcohol may be used instead of Brandy. one galon
Take of the best coniac brandy 4th proof
put it in a bottle and add 3/4 of a tb of
Gum myrrh fine one oz of Cayenne fine
Shake well for 3 or 5 days & it is fit for use

Vegetable Bitters

To make one Junk bottle full. Take of
poplar bark & the leaves & flowers of
thoroughwort ā ā. Enough for about one
quart of Strong tea add about one 1/4 as
much wormwood. Put them into an erthan
vessel & pour boiling water to them boil
them awhile to get out the Strength —
Take 1/2 oz babery bark of the root dried &
pounded fine. Put this into a bowl & add
one teaspoonfull of Cayenne & one table
spoonfull of Sugar. Pour this into the
bowl & Stir the whole together & when
cool add one gill of Brandy or Gin
put all into a Junk bottle, Shake with
it a few times & the bitters are fit for use

Good for Jaundice loss of Appetite Indigestion pain in
the Stomach & bowells caustiveness &c &c

Good for pain in bowels, very hot

Compound Tincture Myrrh Alias No 6.

Alcohol may be used instead of brandy.
Take one of the best cognac brandies, one gallon, 4th proof, put it in a bottle and add ¾ of a ℔[9][pound] of gum myrrh fine, one oz of cayenne fine. Shake well for 5 or 6 days and it is fit for use.

Vegetable Bitters

To make one junk bottle full. Take of poplar bark and the leaves of flowers of thoroughwort[10], enough for about one quart of strong tea, add about one ¼ as much wormwood. Put them into an earthen vessel and pour boiling water to them. Boil them awhile to get out the strength. Take ½ ounce bayberry[11] bark of the root, dried and pounded fine. Put this into a bowl and add one teaspoonful of cayenne and one table spoonful of sugar. Pour this into the bowl and stir the whole together and when cool add one gill[12] of brandy or gin. Put all into a drink bottle, shake it a few times and the bitters are fit for use. Good for jaundice, loss of appetite, indigestion, pain in the stomach and bowels, causativeness.

---

9   pound
10   Eupatorium is a genus of flowering plants in the aster family
11   Bayberry is an upright-rounded, dense shrub
12   Half a cup or 4 fluid ounces

4

Vegetable Ointment

Take one Gallon of neats foot oil and one lb of the bark of the root of bitter Sweet dried & pounded fine ½ lb of camomile pounded & one oz of Cayenne do with on quart of the best Coniac Brandy Stir these together & Simmer over a Slow fire one day. After this Strain off the Oil & add 2 oz Spts Terpentine to each lb of the ointment. This ointment is for all outward applications Such as Calluses Swellings bruises Sprains tightness of the Sinews or Stifness of the Joints &c &c

Vegetable Syrup for Disentary

Take one lb of poplar bark pounded fine one lb of Babery bark do one lb of Gum myrrh do 7 lb of Loaf Sugar 3 Gal of Spring water one Gal of 4 proof Brandy put all these into an iron & let them boil about half hour Strain of the liquor when cool

Vegetable Ointment

Take one gallon of neat's-foot oil[13], add one ℔ [pound] of the bark of the root of bittersweet[14] dried and pounded ½ ℔ [pound] of chamomile pounded and one ounce of cayenne do with one quart of the best cognac brandy. Stir these together and simmer over a slow fire one day. After this strain off the gel and add 2 ounces spirits of turpentine to each ℔ [pound] of the ointment. This ointment is for all outward applications such as calluses, swellings, bruises, sprains, tightness of the sinews or stiffness of the joints.

Vegetable Syrup for Dysentery

Take one pound of poplar bark pounded fine, one ℔ [pound] of bayberry bark, do one ℔ [pound] of Quin myrrh.[15] do 7 ℔ [pound] of loaf sugar, 3 gal of spring water, one gallon of 4 proof brandy. Put all these into an iron and let them boil about half hour. Strain off the liquor when cool and

---

13 Neatsfoot oil is a yellow oil rendered and purified from the shin bones and feet (but not the hooves) of cattle.
14 Woody nightshade
15 Commiphora, an aromatic resin

& put it in bottles Corked tight
& it is fit for use take about one
wine glass full at a time 3 or 4 times
a day as the disorder may require for
children about half as much as for
a grown person &c &c

Worm Syrup

Aloes ℥ß Assofœtida ʒß Chelone
Glabra ℥iv boil the Glabra to one
quart add the Aloes & fœtida &
a quart of Molases - Dose for a
child a tea Spoonfull every half
hour untill it operates as physic —
which brings away worms & Slimy matter

Dysentary

Good vinegar & as much Salt as will
Disolve - add one table Spoonfull to 3
of hot water & let it be taken by table
Spoonfull doses at a time as often
as can be Swallowed every 2 hours
untill it Operates as physic &c

& put it in bottles corked tight. It is fit for use. Take about one wine glass full at a time 3 or 4 times a day as the disorder may require. For children about half as much as for a grown person.

Worm Syrup

Aloes 7ʒ[16][ʒ=ounce] Asafetida[17] ʒss [ʒ=ounce] Chelone Glabra[18] ʒiv [ʒ=ounce] boil the Glabra to one quart add the aloes and foetida[19] and a quart of molasses. Dose for a child: a teaspoonful every half hour until it operates as a physic—which brings away worms and sling mater.

Dysentery

Good vinegar and as much salt as will dissolve. Add one tablespoonful to 3 of hot water and let it be taken by tablespoonful doses at a time as often as can be swallowed every 2 hours until it operates as a physic.

---

16   Apothecaries ounce, https://en.wikipedia.org/wiki/Apothecaries%27_system
17   a Eurasian plant of the parsley family
18   white turtlehead
19   wild maracuja, bush passion fruit

Cough Emulsion

Pulverise or bruise Wild or indian turnip in a fresh State with Loaf Sugar one part of the root with 3 of Sugar beat in a morter in till perfectly united & one of the Strongest Sulution Gum Arabic & the Same of Spermacetia & mix again Add to the above one part of the powdered root of Stilles Foetides & one half part Lobelia mix all & keep in a tight vessel <u>Doce</u> a Spoonfull at bedtime & 2 or 3 times a day &c &c

Sore Eyes

Sal ammoniac gr x, Acetate plumbj (or Sugar Lead) gr v Zinci Sulphas (or white vitrol) gr v tinc Opium drops 100 aqua purae (or pure water) ʒ vi mix fit for use &c &c

Cough Emulsion

Pulverize or bruise wild or Indian turnip in a fresh state with loaf sugar, one part of the root with 3 of sugar, beat in a mortar until perfectly united and one of the strongest solution Gum Arabic and the same of spermaceti[20] and mix again. Add to the above one part of the powdered root of Stoidis Foetidus[21] and one-half part lobelia. Mix all and keep in a tight vessel. Dose: a spoonful at bedtime and 2 or 3 times a day.

Sore Eyes

Sal ammoniac 10 grain[22], Acetate plumby (or sugar lead[23]) 5 grain, ℥mci [℥=ounce] sulfurs (or white vitriol) 5 grain, tincture Opium drops 100 agua purae (or pure water) ℥vi mix fit for use.

---

20 a white waxy substance produced by the sperm whale
21 Perhaps stinking hellebore
22 A grain is 0.065 of a gram or 1/7000 of a pound
23 A poison

Lees Pill

Aloes ℥x ii Scammony ℥vi
Gamboge ℥iv White Helebore ℥viii Jalap
℥iii Calomel ℥v Pill with ext Mandrake. A good physic in all cases where bilious physic is needed

Quick Pill No 1

Gamboge gr xx Aloes xx Colocinth xx
Calomel xxx Scammony xx unite
a little oil or essence peppermint
with ext Mandrake to pill with

Ague Pill

Cayenne Quinine Opium Alum
Bloodroot each one ℥i ext beef
Gall Sufficient to pill with

X Ague pill

Quinine grs x ℞ ♄ ♂ ♀ ☉ grs v ♃ vi
xv African Cayenne grs xv Mix all
well in a wedgewood morter for 15

Lees Pill

Aloes ℥xii [℥=ounce], Scammony[24] ℥vi, Gamboge[25] ℥iv, White Hellebore[26] ℥viii, Salep[27] ℥iii, Calomel[28] ℥v, Pill with extra mandrake[29]. A good physic in all cases where a bilious physic is needed.

Quick Pill No 1

Gamboge grain xx, Aloes xx, Colocynth[30] xx, Calomel xxx, Scammony xx, unite a little oil or essence peppermint with extract mandrake to pill with.

Ague[31] Pill

Cayenne, quinine, opium, alum, bloodroot, each one ℥i [℥=ounce] extract beef gall sufficient to pill with

Ague Pill

Quinine grains x, arsenic[32] grains v, opium[33] xv, African cayenne grains xv Mix all well in a wedge wood mortar for 15

---

24 a plant of the morning glory family
25 Resin of the gamboge tree
26 An herb that was used historically in Rome as a poison
27 a flour made from the tubers of the orchid genus *Orchis*
28 a white powder used as a purgative and a fungicide
29 a Mediterranean plant of the nightshade family
30 a tropical Old-World climbing plant of the gourd family
31 malaria
32 Translated from code on page 1
33 Translated from code

8

minutes so that the x t ϙ ϑ ⅋ may be compleetly mixed with the other articles and pill as little as will suffise of the ext of burdock root or top Dose If the fits come on every day give a pill every hour if every other day a pill may be given every 2 hours if the stomach is much loded with bile or the patient often enclines to vomit give a gentle Emetic of eagual parts Lobelia or Ipicac alone at all events move the bowels with some gentle Physic. N.B. The above is to be mixed and divided into twenty Pills

For Cornes

Disolve Saleratus strong apply a piece of Sponge or a little piece of Cotton often & it will distroy it

Palmonary Mixture

Take 1/3 infusion Slippery Elm or flax Seed hot Add 2 or 3 lemons slised 1/3 Liqurice past Sufficient Sugar

minutes that the arsenic[34] may be completely mixed with the other articles and pill as little as will suffice of the extract of the burdock root or top. Dose: If the fits come on every day, give a pill every hour. If every other day, a pill may be given every 2 hours. If the stomach is much loaded with bile or the patient often inclines to vomit give a gentle emetic of equal parts lobelia or ipecac alone. At all events move the bowels with the same gentle physic. W.B. The above is to be mixed and divided into twenty pills.

For Corns

Dissolve Saleratus[35] strong, apply a piece of sponge or a little piece of cotton often and it will destroy it.

Pulmonary Mixture

Take 1ʒ [ʒ=ounce] infusion slippery elm or flaxseed hot add 2 or 3 lemons sliced 1ʒ [ounce] licorice paste sufficient sugar

---

34 Translated from code
35 Sodium bicarbonate (or sometimes potassium bicarbonate)

Candy to form a Syrup Simmer a few minutes over a Slow fire Strain & when cold add tinc Lobelia 1℥ Tinc blood root 1℥ Tinc Skunk Cabbage 1℥ Tinc balsom Tolu 1℥ or Syrup of Hourhoun 1℥ Doee from a table Spoonfull to a small wine glass 3 or 4 times a day

X   Venerial. Alias DX 9
Piper Cubebia Canadee Balsam
& Bolsom Copebia eaqual parts made into a paste & take the Size of a Common large bean three times a day

Spruice Beer
½ Gal Molasses 2℥ of Ground Ginger a little ext or oil of Spruice ten Gal of water (In common within a bour blood warm) & in part of it a few hops Should be boiled & Strained If very hot wither add one pt of yeast ferment in an open tub Scum & bottle or put in a Keg for Draft (Spruice Beer)

candy to form a syrup. Simmer a few minutes over a slow fire. Strain and when cold add tincture of lobelia 1ʒ [ounce], tincture bloodroot[36] 1ʒ [ounce], tincture skunk cabbage[37] 1ʒ, [ounce] tincture balsam tolu[38] 1ʒ [ounce] or syrup of horehound 1ʒ [ounce]. Dose: from a table spoonful to a small wine glass 3 or 4 times a day.

Venereal Alias Clap[39]

Piper lobelia[40], Canada balsam[41], and balsam copaiba[42] equal parts made into a paste and take the size of a common large bean three times a day.

Spruce Beer

½ gallon molasses, 2ʒ [ounce] of ground ginger, a little extract or oil of spruce, ten gallons of water (in common weather about blood warm). One part of it, a few tops, should be boiled and strained. If very hot weather add one pint of yeast, ferment in a jar or tub, scum x bottles or put in a keg for draft. (Spruce beer)

---

36 *Sanguinaria canadensis*
37 Indian Wax Paper, used for cramps, blood purifier, and kidney cleanser
38 a sap-like substance that comes from the Myroxylon balsamum tree
39 Translated from code on page 1
40 Lobelia inflata, an anitispasmodic, respiratory stimulant, relaxant, emetic and euphoriant.
41 Balm of Gilead is used for burns, sores, cuts, tumors, heart and chest pains, cancer, inflammation, colds, coughs, warts, wounds and pain relief.
42 Copaifera officinalis

Diarhoea

Rhubarb ʒ 1 Brandy ʒ 1 Paragoric ʒ 1 Loaf Sugar Sufficient to render it Agreeable Saleratus one drachm peppermint water half pint —

Hiera Picra

Aloes 1 ℔ Ginger 1/4 ℔ Winter or Canella bark 1/4 ℔ Pulv each Seperate and mix all together one oz in a pt of Spirits —

Cough Drops

Sweet oil 1 pt Raw flax Seed Oil 1/2 pt honey 1/2 pt Spts Terpentine 1 oz Balsom of life 1 oz Liquorice Ball one oz all to be Simmered untill well mixed Doce from 10 to 60 Drops Good for Colds coughs &c

New Vegetable Physic

Culvers Root mandrake root Iris versicolar Cream tarter Ginger of each one drachm to be taken in hot water Sweetened to your taste to be repeated every 2 or 3 hours
Add Jalup ʒ 1 &c

Diarrhea

Rhubarb ℥I [℥=ounce], Brandy ℥i, Paregoric[43] ℥i, Loaf Sugar sufficient to render it agreeable, Saleratus one drachm, peppermint water half pint.

Hiera Picra[44]

Aloes 1 ℔ [pound], Ginger ¼ ℔ [pound], Winter or Canella[45] bark ¼ ℔ [pound], pulverize separately and mix all together one ounce in a pint of spirits.

Cough Drops

Sweet oil 1 pint, raw flax seed oil ½ pint, honey ½ pint, spirits turpentine 1 ounce, balsam of life 1 ounce, licorice ball 1 ounce, all to be simmered until well mixed. Dose: from 10 to 50 drops, good for colds, coughs.

New Vegetable Physic

Culver's root[46], mandrake root, Iris versicolor[47], cream tartar, ginger, of each one drachm to be taken in hot water sweetened to your taste to be repeated every 2 or 3 hours. Add Salep[48] ℥i [℥=ounce]

---

43 camphorated tincture of opium
44 A warming cathartic medicine made from aloes and canella
45 White cinnamon
46 *Veronicastrum virginicum*
47 Northern blue flag
48 A flour made from the tubers of the orchid genus *Orchis*

Spruce Beer

Water ten Gall Mollases 3 quarts Ginger one tea cup full Alspice 2 & ½ oz yeast ½ pt hops Ginger Alspice boiled till all Settled mollases & Spruce Disolved in a pail added to the rest Strain all into a cask Stir in the yeast when fermentation ceases Bung up fit for use &c

Itch Ointment

Sulphuric Acid ʒiii oil of Terpentine ʒiv Olive oil xʒ mix (Infalable)

Compound Balsom

Bolsom fir ʒii do Tolu ʒi British oil ʒi White Pine Terpentine ʒi huney ʒii mix Doce 12 to 16 drops for pains in the chest or caused by a Strain from a weak Stomach

Ginger Beer

Spruce Beer

Water ten gallons, molasses 3 quarts, ginger one tea cup full, allspice 2½ ounce, yeast ½ pint, hops, ginger allspice boiled till all settled, molasses and spruce dissolved in a pail added to the rest. Strain all into a cask, stir in the yeast when fermentation ceases. Bring up fit for use.

Itch Ointment

Sulfuric acid ʒiii [ʒ=ounce], oil of turpentine ʒiv, olive oil ʒx mix (Infallible)[49]

Compound Balsam

Balsam fir ʒii [ʒ=ounce], do Tolu[50] ʒi, British oil ʒi, White Pine turpentine ʒi, honey ʒii, mix. Dose: 12 to 40 drops for pains in the chest or caused by a strain from a weak stomach.

Ginger Beer

---

49 Probably not as this is crossed off...
50 a fragrant brown balsam obtained from a South American tree

Pox Medicine

Bitter Sweet & flax seed oil simered together. Black root Sarseparlia prickly ash a a parts Boil to a Strong tee add as much Spirits as will keep it from Soring Certin cure for pox from Nathan Harlon

Cure for Gravel

Take 5 egg Shells dry & pulverize put into one quart of boiling water drink all in one day & the next day drink out quart Slippery Elm tee

Good for the Itch

Take Black Root 2 oz Boil Strong in a pot or Iron Kettle wash freely & drink do

Ague Bitters

Put in three half pints of good Brandy or other good Spirit one oz of Golden Seal Pulv half oz good Composition ½ oz Blood root Dose all the Stomach will bear 3 or 4 times a day

p o x Medicine

Bittersweet and flaxseed oil simmered together. Blackroot sarsaparilla, prickly ash of each parts. Boil to a strong tea add as much spirits as will keep it from (?). Certain cure for p o x[51] from Nathan Harlon.

Cure For Gravel[52]

Take 5 egg shells dry and pulverize, put into one quart of boiling water. Drink all in one day and the next day drink one quart slippery elm tea.

Good for the Itch

Take black root 2 oz, boil strong in a pot or iron kettle, wash freely and drink do.

Ague Bitters

Put in three half pints of good Brandy or other good Spirit, one ounce of Golden Seal[53] pulverized, half ounce of good Composition, ½ ounce of bloodroot.[54] Dose: all the stomach will bear 3 or 4 times a day.

---

51 This translates from code.
52 Kidney stones
53 Goldenseal is an herb. The dried root is used to make medicine.
54 Bloodroot is used to cause vomiting, empty the bowels, and reduce tooth pain.

For bots & Belly ache in Horses

Give Nux Vomica in whiskey or water 1 pt
It will cure either bots or Chills in 30 minutes
For belly ache. Give 4 Gallon weak lie & pour
Salt water on the loins Sure Cure

Itch Ointment
Carefully melt your butter rosin together add
the terpentine & lastly the precipitate work
all well together. Use no Sulphur at the time
of using the ointment. Be carefull to melt
your butter & rosin well together in the first place
  Fresh Butter one lb
  Red Precipitate 2 oz
  Rosin or Burgsh 2 oz
  Spts Terpentine 2 oz

Medical or Root Beer
Sassafras root (Rad. Sasafras) qs
Burdock Root (Arctium Lappa) qs
Wild Cherry Bark or Root (Prinos Virginiana) qs
Root of Black Alder (Prinos Verticillatus) qs
Make a Strong decoction by Boiling several

For bots[55] and Bellyache in Horses

Give Nux Vomica[56] in whiskey or water 1 pint. It will cure either bots or cholic in 30 minutes. For bellyache give ½ gallon weak lye and pour salt water on the loins. Sure cure.[57]

Itch Ointment[58]

Carefully melt your butter, rosin together, add the turpentine and lastly the precipitate work all well together. Use no sulphur at the time of using the ointment. Be careful to melt your butter and rosin well together in the first place.

Fresh Butter one pound
Red Precipitate[59] 2 ounces
Rosin or Burg Pitch 2 ounces
Spirits Turpentine 2 ounces

Medical or Root Beer

Sassafras root (*Rad. Sassafras*) gp
Burdock root (*Arctium Lappa*) gp
Wild Cherry Bark or Root (*Prinos Virginiana*) gp
Root of Black Alder (*Prinos Verticillatus*) gp
Make a Strong decoction by boiling several

---

55 Internal parasites
56 Nux vomica is a tree. The seed is used to make medicine. Nux vomica contains strychnine and brucine, two deadly chemicals.
57 Maybe not…it is crossed off
58 Also crossed off
59 Mercuric oxide

hours Strain Sweeten well with mollasses or honey then add when it is Blood warm Sufficient yeast to foment it. In a short time or as Soon as it Commences fomentation it is fit for use. This may be taken freely as a diet drink. It is very plesent & Excelent to prevent disease & keep the Sistem in a helthy State and it is Gratefull & Cooling in all kinds of favers &c

---

Rhumatic Limment
Alchohol   15 Gallons
Oil of Wormwood   2 lb
Oil of Origanum   3 lb
Oil of Sasafras   1 lb
Casteal Soap   1½ lb
Oil Vitriol   ½ lb
Capsicum Anum   1½ lb
Beef Gall   ¼ Gal

Mix Stir often for 10 days fit for use

Add Discretionary ½
Gine Files
Gum Cemph
Jf.o Terpentime

Black Salve
Sugar Lead ℥ij Grined well togther put into
Litharge ℥j a kettle with half lb lard

hours, strain, sweeten well with molasses or honey, then add when it is blood warm Sufficient yeast to ferment it. In a short time or as soon as it commences fermentation, it is fit for use. This may be taken freely as a diet drink. It is very pleasant and excellent to prevent disease and keep the system in a healthy state, and it is grateful and cooling in all kinds of flavors.

Rheumatic Liniment

Add discretionary
Tincture Flies[60]
Gum Camphor
Spirits of turpentine

Alcohol 16 gallons
Oil of Wormwood[61] 2 ℔ [pound]
Oil of Origanum[62] 3 ℔ [pound]
Oil of Sassafras[63] 1 ℔ [pound]
Castile Soap[64] 1½ ℔ [pound]
Oil Vitriol[65] ½ ℔ [pound]
Capsicum Annum[66] 1½ ℔ [pound]
Beef Gall[67] 1½ gallon

Mix, stir often for 10 days, fit for use

Black Salve

Sugar Lead ℥ijs [℥=ounce], Grind well together, put into Litharge ℥j a kettle with half ℔ [pound] lard.

---

60 Cantharidin powder, Spanish Fly, a deadly Viagra of the past
61 Artemisia absinthium
62 a genus of herbaceous perennials and subshrubs in the family Lamiaceae
63 Currently banned in the U.S. as a carcinogen
64 Castile Soap is a plant based soap made from vegetable oil such as olive, coconut, palm, or any other plant based oil rather than from animal fat.
65 Sulfuric acid
66 A chili pepper
67 The gall (bile) of cattle is prepared for medical purposes by simply evaporating it at a moderate heat, in a shallow pan.

Bring to a boiling heat & Stir all the time until it turns black take off the fire & it is done. If you wish it harder you can add one oz or less or more of melted Beeswax while the Salve is yet hot from the fire. Good in all Cuts burns Scalds old Sores &c &c

Best Adhesive Plaster

Eaqual parts of rosin burgundy pitch White Diacylum united together forms one of the most adhesive plasters known for heeling together or uniting cuts or for whatever use adhesive plaster may be needed &c

---

℞ Fever & Ague
White Vitrol   Sulph Zinc   Ɔ i
Red Pepper   Capsicum   Ɔ ii
Quinine   Quinine   Ɔ i
Salt of Black Pepper Piperine Ɔ ii
Polen of Hops   Lupuline   Ɔ ii

Ext of Taraxicum. Ext dandelion, qs to make 100 pills
If the Pills are found not Sufficiently powerfull add
Ɔ i more to the Quinine & Sulph Zinc which makes
2 Scruples each of all the articles

Give one Emetic then a pill Every hour between Paroxisms
Chicago April 16, 34

Bring to a boiling heat and stir all the time until it turns black. Take off the fire and it is done. If you wish it harder, you can add one ounce or less or more of melted Beeswax while the salve is yet hot from the fire. Good in all cuts, burns, scalds, old sores.

Best Adhesive Plaster

Equal parts of resin burgundy pitch, white diacylum[68] united together forms one of the best adhesive plasters known for healing together or uniting cuts or whatever use adhesive plaster may be needed.

Rx Fever and Ague

Give an emetic then a pill every hour between paroxysms. Chicago, April 16, 44

White Vitriol	Sulphur Zinc $\ni i$[69] [$\ni$ = scruple]
Red Pepper	Capsicum $\ni ii$
Quinine	Quinine $\ni i$
Salts of Black Pepper	Piperine $\ni ii$
Pollen of Hops	Lupulin $\ni ii$

Extract of Taraxacum, extract of dandelion, gp to make two pills. If the pills are found not sufficiently powerful add $\ni I$ [$\ni$=scruple] more to the quinine and Sulphur zinc, which makes scruples each of all of the articles.

---

68 Possibly diatomaceous earth
69 The $\ni$ symbol is for scruple 1.296 grams

16   I have got this in my Large book
                                Wallace
              Ammenagogue

℞   Black Cohush   3 oz
         Secale Cormutum   4 oz Spurdrye
Steep the above in 3 quarts of Proof Spirits
Doce a tea spoonfull of the tine in a cup of
flax seed or Slippery Elm tea 3 or 4 times a
day to act as an Ammenagogue & more frequently to produce abortion. After taking this
medicine extreme care must be had not to take
cold as it would produce Serious Consequences as
the med has a direct action on the uterine vessels
produces a relaxed State of the womb
and its appendages &c

℞   X For Gonorrhoea or Clap
Take one tea Spoonfull of Oil Sassafras
one & a half oz No 6 one & a half oz Balsam
Copaiba half oz Spts Nitre Dulc fill up
the viol which must hold 8 oz with the
Alterative below Doce one tea Spoonfull 3 times
a day   Goac wood   2 lb
          Pipsisaway   1 1/2 lb
         Burdock Seeder Root 1/2 lb

I have got this in my Large Book—Wallace[70]

Emmenagogue[71]

Black Cohosh[72] 3 oz
Secale Cornutum[73] 4 oz Spurge

Steep the above in 3 quarts of proof spirits.
Dose: a teaspoonful if the time in a cup of flaxseed or slippery elm tea 3 or 4 times a day to act as an emmenagogue and more frequently to produce abortion. After taking this medicine extreme care must be had not to take cold as it would produce serious consequences, as the med has a direct action on the uterine vessels, produces a relaxed state of the womb and its appendages.

Rx For Gonorrhea or Clap

Take one tea spoonful of oil sassafras, one and a half oz No. 6, one and a half oz Balsam Copaiba[74], half oz spirits Nitre[75] ??, fill up the vial which must hold 8 oz with the Alternative below.
Dose: one teaspoonful three times a day.

Guaiac[76] Wood 2 ℔ [pound]
Pipsissewa[77] 1½ ℔ [pound]
Burdock Lower Root ½ ℔ [pound]

---

70 Lois Hale Reid has this Large Book
71 Herbs that stimulate blood flow in the pelvic area and uterus
72 also called black bugbane, black snakeroot, baneberry, or fairy candle
73 Ergot
74 Copaiba balsam is a sap-like substance (oleoresin).
75 Ethyl nitrite
76 Most likely oil from the palo santo tree (Bulnesia sarmientoi)
77 AKA Bitter Winter, Bitter Wintergreen, Chimaphila

Sarseparilla 1 ℔
Blue Cohosh ¼ ℔

Step in hot water over night Slow boil one hour Strain add more water let Stand in a hot place 3 or 4 hours boil on hour an Strain & So proceed as above untill the Strength is all extracted. Strain all & reduce to 15 quarts add 2 gal Sugar House molasses & 2 quart Hol Gin Essence Sassafras 2 oz Doce wine Glass 3 times a day
Best medicine now in use by all obts &c

My Emetic

Emetic Doctor ix White Helebore ℈iv grs xv Mandrake ʒvj Lobelia of the Seed ʒiiij Pulverize all well togather Doce From Six to fifteen grs repeted every fifteen or twenty minutes untill three doses may be taken & if the three doses do not operate give Great quantities thurroughwort or Camomile tea & a doce or two of Saleratus & warm water & Stimulate with Capsicum Anum or Cayenne Soac the feet &c

Sarsaparilla[78] 1 ℔ [pound]
Blue Cohosh[79] ½ ℔ [pound]

Steep in hot water overnight slow boil one hour, strain, add more water, let stand in a hot place 3 or 4 hours, boil an hour and strain, and to proceed as above until the strength is all extracted. Strain all, reduce to 16 quarts, add 2 gal sugar house molasses and 2 quarts hot gin, essence sassafras, 2 oz.
Dose: wine glass 3 times a day.
Best medicine now in use by all able.

My Emetic[80]

Emetic Tartar[81] ix, White Hellebore[82] ℈iv grs xv [℈=scruple], Mandrake[83] ℥vji [℥=ounce], Lobelia[84] ℥jjjj. Pulverize all well together. Dose: From six to fifteen grs repeated every fifteen or twenty minutes until three doses may be taken. If the three doses do not operate, give great quantities thoroughwort[85] or chamomile[86] tea and a dose or two of Saleratus[87] and warm water. Stimulate with capsicum annum or cayenne. Soak the feet.

---

78 Sarsaparilla and sassafras contain safrole, a compound recently banned by the FDA due to its carcinogenic effects.
79 Caulophyllum, not considered a safe plant.
80 Note that this is crossed off
81 Antimony potassium tartarate, a poison
82 A poison used to make medicine
83 One of the uses of mandrake is to trigger vomiting.
84 Listed as a potentially toxic herb.
85 Eupatorium serotinum
86 Considered a safe plant
87 Sodium bicarbonate

18 Take 3 carrots, grate them fine, into a vessel, cover them with lard; boil them thoroughly, strain & add sufficient of beeswax to make a paste —

Diarrhoea or Bowel disease
Burn Rhubarb powder in an iron vessel, stirring it until it blackens, then smother it in a covered jar, it looses two thirds its weight by incineration and is nearly tasteless — it may be given in port wine, or milk and water, after 2 or 3 doses pains quickly subside and the bowels return to their natural state

Carbonated Beer

℞ 60. lbs sugar
   4 lbs Tartaric Acid
   4 Gallons Strong Beer
   1 oz Oil Lemon. mix

Add Soda when you wish to use it

Ginger Beer

℞. Take lump or loaf sugar 1½ lb of Cream Tarter ½ oz. Bruised Ginger one oz. Boiling Water one gallon forment 24 hours with yeast a bottle in rate like

Take 3 carrots, grate them fine into a vessel. Cover them with lard; boil them thoroughly, strain and add sufficient of beeswax to make a paste.

Diarrhea or Bowel Disease

Burn rhubarb powder in an iron vessel, stirring it until it blackens, then smother it in a covered jar. It loses two thirds of its weight by incineration and is nearly tasteless—it may be given in port wine or milk and water, after 2 or 3 doses pains quickly subside and the bowels return to their natural state.

Rx Carbonated Beer

60 ℔ [pounds] sugar
4 ℔ [pounds] tartaric acid
4 gallons strong beer
1 oz oil lemon mix
Add soda when you wish to use it.

Ginger Beer

Rx Take lump or loaf sugar ½ ℔ [pound] of cream tartar ½ oz. Bruise ginger one oz. Boiling water one gallon, ferment 24 hours with yeast a bottle if raw like.

Pill Pargantia

℞ Aloes ʒi" Colocynth ʒi'
Gamboge ʒi' White Helebore ʒi'
Soap ʒi' Emetic tart 15 grs
You can use two scruple of Gamboge instead of ʒi, and 10 grs of Emetic tart and they will not cause so much sickness at the stomach & will act a little more slowly

---

Ice Cream } Ice cream can be made of all cream, or of new milk, or, a part cream & part milk, a part each does well „ To Six quarts add one & half lb Loaf, or lump, or good Muscovada Sugar,, 1/3 of an oz of Essence of Lemon or to suit your taste. To every quart of the milk add 4 eggs, Vanilla bean can be used, one ~~bean is~~ third of a bean is sufficient for Six quarts, cut or pound it, tye it up in a rag boil it in a little of the milk press it out through the rag & add to the rest of it, turn the pail round part of the time & often and constantly scrape the

Pill Purgantia[88]

Aloes ℥ii [℥=ounce], Colocynth[89] ʒi,
Gamboge[90] ʒi. White Hellebore[91] ʒi,
Soup ʒi, Emetic tart[92] 15 grains

You can use two scruples of Gamboge instead of ʒi, and 10 grains of Emetic tart and they will cause so much sickness at the stomach and will act a little more slowly.

Ice Cream

Ice cream can be made of all cream, or of new milk, or a part cream and part milk, apart, each does well. To six quarts add one and one half ℔ [pound] loaf, or lump, or good Muscovado Sugar[93], 1/3 of an oz of essence of lemon or to suit your taste. To every quart of the milk add 4 eggs. Vanilla bean can be used, one third of a bean is sufficient for six quarts. Cut or pound it, tie it up in a rag boil it in a little of the milk, press it out through the rag and add it to the rest of it. Turn the pail round part of the time often and constantly scrape the

---

88 Makes you throw up
89 Contains cucurbitacins which are extremely irritating to mucous membranes.
90 Resin from the evergreen Clusiaceae family
91 A poison used to make medicine
92 Antimony potassium tartrate, a poison
93 Unrefined cane sugar that contains natural molasses.

20 Cream as it cools on the side of the pail down to the centre of the pail — First saw a barrel in two & use for the out side vessel, then get a new tub to fill the out side one within three inches put pounded charcoal on the bottom of the out side tub & fill all round the inside tub between that and the out side one = next put the ice on the botton of the inside tub and all round the pail with a little salt & add salt by littles until the cream is frose, it requires a quart of salt to six quarts or a pail full to freeze it = the tin pail must have a cover & be made nine inches across the top & nine & half deep —

Corn Meal Cakes

Breakfast cakes can be made in the following manner as good as victorea will ever say, from cincinnati Kiln dried corn meal. Mix 2 quarts corn meal at night with water & a little yast & salt just thin enough to stir easy. In the morning stir in 3 or 4 Eggs a little saleratus & a cup of sour milk so as to leave it thin enough to pour out of a pan. Bake

cream as it cools on the side of the pail down into the center of the pail.

First, saw a barrel in two and use for the outside vessel, then fit a new tub to fill the outside one within three inches. Put pounded charcoal on the bottom of the outside tub and fill all round the inside tub between that and the outside one—next put the ice on the bottom of the inside tub and all round the pail with a little salt by littles until the cream is froze. It requires a quart of salt to six quarts on a pail full to freeze it = the tin pail must have a cover and be made nine inches across and nine and a half deep.

Corn Meal Cakes

Breakfast cakes can be made in the following manner as good as Victoria will ever enjoy from Cincinnati. Kiln dried corn meal. Mix 2 quarts corn meal at night with water and a little yeast and salt, just thin enough to stir easy. In the morning, stir 3 or 4 eggs, a little Saleratus[94] and a cup of sour milk so as to leave it thin enough to pour out of a pan. Bake

---

94 Sodium bicarbonate

three quarters of an hour and you will have a rich honey comb cake

Genuine Whigs
2 tbs of flour 8 oz Butter 8 oz sugar 6 Eggs one pt milk raise with yeast make them Before dinner and by Tea time they will be ready to Bake

Cookies
Take 12 oz of sugar ½ lb of Butter ½ pt milk 2 spoonfulls of pearlash

Another
Take 2 Tea cups of cream 1 of sugar 1 Tea spoonfull of pearlash & 2 Eggs

Wafers
One lb of flour 8 oz of Butter 6 Eggs 3¼ lb of sugar 1 oz of caraway seed

Jumbles
5 tbs of flour 2 tbs of sugar 1 lb of butter 6 Eggs roll them out in sugar

Three quarters of an hour and you will have a rich honey comb cake.

Genuine Whigs

2 ℔ [pounds] of flour, 8 oz Butter, 8 oz sugar, one pint milk raise with yeast, make them before dinner and by tea time they will be ready to bake.

Cookies

Take 12 oz of sugar, ½ oz. of butter, ½ pint milk, 2 spoonfuls of pearlash[95].

Another

Take 2 tea cups of cream, 1 of sugar, two spoonfuls of pearlash and 2 eggs.

Wafers

One ℔ [pound] of flour, 8 oz of butter, 6 eggs, ¾ ℔ [pound] of sugar, 1 oz or caraway seed.

Jumbles

5 ℔ [pounds] of flour, 2 ℔ [pound] of sugar, 1 ℔ [pound] of butter, 6 eggs, roll them out in sugar.

---

95 chemically known as potassium carbonate K_2CO_3

Cookies

3 lbs of flour 12 oz of Butter 12 oz sugar
2 tee spoonfulls of perlash disolve the
sugar in a half pt of water. Spice

Nut Cake

7 lbs of flour 2 lbs of Sugar 12 oz
of Butter yeast wet with new milk
Eggs if you plase + Cinnamon +

Muffins

1 lb of flour one pt of milk 8 eggs
Beat them well put in as much yeast
as you think will raise them. Bake
them as soon as you can

Number Cake

One tea cup full of ~~flour~~ Butter 2 tea
cups full of sugar 3 tea cups full of flour
4 Eggs nutmeg & Brandy

Rusk

5 lbs of flour ½ a lb of butter 12 oz sugar

Cookies

3 ℔ [pounds] of flour, 12 oz of Butter, 12 oz sugar, 2 tea spoonfuls of pearlash, dissolve the sugar in a half pint of water. Spice.

Nut Cake

7 ℔ [pounds] of flour, 2 ℔ [pounds] of sugar, 12 oz of butter, yeast wet with new milk, eggs if you please, cinnamon.

Muffins

1 ℔ [pound] of flour, one pint of milk, 8 eggs. Beat them well, put in as much yeast as you think will raise them. Bake them as soon as you can.

Number Cake

One tea cup full of Butter, 2 tea cups full of sugar, 3 tea cups full of flour, 4 eggs, nutmeg & brandy

Rusks

5 ℔ [pounds] of flour, ½ a ℔ [pound] of butter, 12 oz sugar.

9 Eggs 1 pt of milk yeast as much as you think Propper

Masure Cake
Take 2 coffee cups of sugar 1 of Butter 1 of Cream 1 Glap of Brandy 1/2 a nutmeg 9 Eggs

Little Cake
1 lb of Butter 1 lb 4 oz of Sugar 1 lb of currants 6 Eggs

Sponge Cake
the yolk of 10 Eggs 1 lb of sugar roll them well together add the whites ofter Yeavering beat them to a froth with 10 oz of flour It ought not to be put in untill Just fore it is put into the oven

Plumb Cake
9 lbs of flour 9 Eggs 3 lbs of sugar 1 pt of yeast 1 spoonfull of rose water spice to your taste and as much milk as will wet it

9 eggs, 1 pint of milk, yeast as much as you think proper.

Measure Cake

Take 2 coffee cups of sugar, 1 of Butter, 1 of cream, glass of Brandy, ½ a nutmeg, 9 eggs

Little Cake

1 ℔ of Butter, 1 ℔ [pound] 4 oz of sugar, 1 ℔ [pound] of currants, 6 eggs

Sponge Cake

The yolk of 10 eggs, 1 ℔ [pound] of sugar, roll them well together, add the whites after having beat them to a froth, with 10 ℥ [ounces] of flour. It ought not to be put in until just before it is put into the oven.

Plum Cake

9 ℔s [pounds] of flour, 9 eggs, 3 ℔s [pounds] of sugar, 1 pint of yeast, 1 spoonful of rose water, spice to your taste and as much milk as will wet it.

Crockers

4 oz of Butter 4 Eggs 1 pt of milk

Ginger Bread

Eaqual quantities of Cream & Molasses a large potion of perlash disolved in sharp vinegar make it hard and put Ginger to your tast

Fruit Cake

2 lbs of flour 2 do of currants 1 & 1/4 of Butter 1 & 1/4 of sugar Sixteen Eggs 1/2 oz nutmeg 3/4 pt wine the same of Brandy

Puff Paste

2 lbs of flour 1 lbs of Butter the whites of 2 Eggs

York Biskit

2 lb 12 oz of flour 6 oz of Butter half a spoonfull of pearlash disolve it in as much milk as will make it hard

Crockers

4 oz of Butter, 4 eggs, 1 pint of milk

Ginger Bread

Equal quantities of cream and molasses, a large portion of pearlash dissolved in sharp vinegar, make it hard and put ginger to your taste.

Fruit Cake

2 ℔s [pounds] of flour, 2 do of currants, 1¼ of Butter, 1¼ of sugar, sixteen eggs, ½ oz nutmeg, ¾ pint wine, the same of brandy.

Puff Paste

2 ℔s [pounds] of flour, 1 ℔ [pound] of butter, the white of 2 eggs

York Biscuit

2 ℔ [pounds] 12 oz of flour, 6 oz of butter, half a spoonful pearlash, dissolve it in as much milk as will make it hard.

Whip Sillabub

one qt of thick cream one gill of wine the Juice of 2 Lemmons in a pound of Loaf sugar pour it into a large pan Then Beat it well & as the froth rises to the top take it off & put it in a glass

Common Loaf Cake

eight quarts of flour 3 lbs & oz of Butter 4 lbs of sugar one gallon of milk one pt of wine one pt of yeast.

Icing for Cake

2 lbs of double refined sugar beat & sift it through a fine sieve put into it a spoonfull of fine starch a penny worth worth of Gum Arabec beat them well together Take the whites of 4 or 5 Eggs beat them well & put in a spoonfull of rose water & a spoonfull of Lemon Juice beat them with your Eggs & put a little in your sugar till you wet it then beat them till your cake is Baked put it on with a Knife

Whip Syllabub

One quart of thick cream, one gill of wine, the juice of 3 lemons, ½ a pound of loaf sugar, pour it into a large pan, then beat it well and as the froth rises to the top, take it off and put it into a glass.

Common Loaf Cake

Eight quarts of flour, 3 tbs [pounds] 8 oz of butter, 4 tbs [pounds] of sugar, one gallon of milk, one pint of wine, one pint of yeast.

Icing for Cake

2 tbs [pounds] of double refined sugar, beat and sift it through a fine sieve, put into it a spoonful of fine starch, a penny was the worth of gum Arabic. Beat them well together. Take the whites of 4 or 5 eggs, beat them well and put in a spoonful of rose water and a spoonful of lemon juice. Beat them with your eggs and put a little in your sugar till you wet it then beat them till your cake is baked. Put it on with a knife.

26)

The real John Bull Pudding

1 lb of flour, 1 do Zante currents, 1 do resins (stoned) 1 do Beef suet cut middling fine 8 yolks & 4 whites of Eggs ½ a nutmeg grated, 1 Tea spoonfull ginger 1 pt sweet milk. Beat the Eggs then put to them half the milk & beat them together & by degrees stir in the flour, then the suet Spice & fruit and as much more of the milk as will mix it well together very thick it will take 4 hours in boiling stew with grated sugar when on the dish

Cookies Again

5 spoons Buttermilk 2 Butter put the above in a tea cup & then fill it up with sugar, make thick Enough to roll with flour add seeds if you like

Harrison Cake

1 lb of sugar ½ butter ¾ of flour 4 eggs, 6 spoons cream, 1 glass wine 1 do Brandy fruit & Orange peel

The Real John Bull Pudding

1 ℔ [pound] of flour, 1 do Zante currants, 1 do raisins (stoned), 1 do beef suet cut middling fine, 8 yolks, and 4 whites of eggs, ½ a nutmeg grated, 1 tea spoonful ginger, 1 pint sweet milk. Beat the eggs then put to them half the milk and beat them together and by degrees stir in the flour, then the suet, spice, and fruit, and as much more of the milk as will mix it well together very thick, it will take 4 hours in boiling stew with grated sugar when on the dish.

Cookies Again

5 spoons buttermilk, 2 butter, put the above in a teacup and then fill it up with sugar, make thick enough to roll with flour, add seeds if you like.

Harrison Cake

1 ℔ [pound] of sugar, ½ butter, ¾ of flour, 4 eggs, 6 spoons cream, glass wine, 1 do brandy, fruit, and ginger peel.

Cream Cake

4 cups flour 3 of sugar 1 oz Butter
1 of Cream 5 Eggs 1 Tea spoon of perlash
rub the Butter & sugar together then add the
rest

Sunderland Pudding

1 pt milk 4 Eggs 7 spoons flour
Eat with suet sauce

Pound Cake

1 lb of flour 1 do of Butter 1 of sugar
10 Eggs or 16 whites of Eggs 1 Glass Brandy
Nutmeg & mace

Kings Cake

1 lb of flour 1 of sugar 1/2 of Butter 8
Eggs 1 Glass brandy 1 do wine
1 lb of raisins & Orange peel

Indelable Ink

Pulverise 1/2 worth of lunar Costic & mix
with 1 table spoonfull of vinegar shake before
using wet the place to be marked with a

Cream Cake

4 cups flour, 3 of sugar, 1 oz Butter, 1 of cream, 5 eggs, 1 tea spoon of pearlash, rub the butter and sugar together then add the rest.

Sunderland Pudding

1 pint milk, 4 eggs, 7 spoons of flour, eat with suet sauce.

Pound Cake

1 ℔ [pound] of flour 1 do of Butter, 1 of sugar, 10 eggs or 16 whites of eggs, 1 glass Brandy, nutmeg, and mace[96].

Kings Cake

1 ℔ [pound] of flour, 1 of sugar, ½ of Butter, 8 eggs, 1 glass brandy, 1 do wine, 1 ℔ [pound] of raisins and orange peel.

Indelible Ink

Pulverize 11 worth of lunar caustic[97] and mix with 1 table spoonful of vinegar. Shake before using. Wet the place to be marked with a

---

96 Mace is a yellowish-brown spice that is derived from the dried lacy coating of the nutmeg seed.
97 Silver nitrate

solution of perlash and water &
smooth with a warm Iron

To Colour Green

1 oz Indigo 6 oz oil vitriol stored one
week & be well shaken every day —
after dying the articles yellow put into the
dye while boiling hot 1 spoonfull of the
above composition to 1 pail full of the dye

Pound Cake will keep 1 year

1 lb of sugar 1 lb of flour 12 Eggs
1 lb of Butter with currents or raisins
& nutmeg or mace & a little cinnamon
& then put on the Icing to your like

Pudding

4 lbs of flour 3 lbs of raisins stoned Beef
suet cut fine 1 lb any kind of spices
boil in a stout cloth Saleratus dissolved
in warm water. do not tie the cloth tight or the
pudding

solution of pearlash and water. Smooth with a warm iron.

To Colour Green

1 oz of Indigo, 6 oz oil vitriol. Stand one week and be well shaken every day—often dying the articles yellow, put into the dye while boiling hot, 1 teaspoonful of the above composition to 1 pail full of the dye.

Pound Cake—will keep 1 year

1 ℔ [pound] of sugar, 1 ℔ [pound] of flour, 12 eggs, 1 [pound] of butter with currants or raisins & nutmeg or mace and a little cinnamon. Then put on the icing to your like.

Pudding

4 ℔s [pounds] of flour 3 ℔s [pounds] of raisins stoned, Beef suet cut fine 1 ℔ [pound] any kind of spices 1 ℥. Boil in a stout cloth, Saleratus[98] dissolved ℥js [℥=ounce] in warm water. Do not tie the cloth tight or the pudding

---

98 Sodium bicarbonate

Birds Nest Pudding

If you wish to make what is called "birds nest pudding," prepare your custard,— Take 8 or 10 plesent apples pare them them & dig out the cores,, but leave them hole; set them in a pudding dish pore your custard over them & bake them about thirty minutes

Gingerbread

1 lb of flour half a lb of Butter & do Sugar rubbed into it 1/2 a lb of sugar great spoonfull of Ginger or more according to the strength of the Ginger a spoonfull of rose water and a hand full of caraway seed well beat up kneeded stiff Enough to roll out and bake on flat pans 20 or 30 minutes

Cider Cake

Is very good to be baked in small loves 1 1/2 lbs of flour 1/2 lb Sugar 1/2 lb Butter 1/2 pt of cider one Teaspoonfull of pearlash & spice to your taste bake untill it turns easely in the pans I should think about 30 minutes

Birds Nest Pudding

If you wish to make what is called "bird's nest pudding," prepare your custard, take 8 or 10 pleasant apples, pare them and dig out the cores, but leave them whole, set them in a pudding dish, pour your custard over them and bake them about thirty minutes.

Gingerbread

1 ℔ [pound] of flour, half a ℔ [pound] of butter, ½ do sugar rubbed into it, ½ a ℔ [pound] of sugar, great spoonful of ginger or more according to the strength of the ginger, a spoonful of rose water and a handful of caraway seed well beat up, kneaded stiff enough to roll out and bake on flat pans 20 or 30 minutes.

Cider Cake

Is very good to be baked in small loaves. 1½ ℔s [pounds] of flour, ½ ℔ [pound] sugar, ½ ℔ [pound] butter, ½ pint of cider, one teaspoonful of pearlash & spice to your taste, bake until it turns easily in the pans. I should think about 30 minutes.

Bread

2 spoonfulls of Cream tarter & mix
dry with one quart of flour then add
three forths of a table spoonfull of super car-
benete of soda mix the whole with sweet
milk & bake immediately

To cure Warts

Aqua Ammoniae Tinc Cantharides
a unifmix if not the warts should be
wet frequently with one of them &
the other Alternately every day

Soft Gingerbread

One & a ½ lbs of flour 12 oz of sugar
8 Eggs Ginger to your taste Pearlash

Cookies

Take 2 lbs of flour 12 oz of sugar
½ lb of Butter ½ pt milk 2 Tea spoonfulls pearlas

French Loaf

1 lb of sugar 1 lb of flour ½ lb Butter ½ a lb

Bread

2 spoonfuls of cream tartar & mix dry with one quart of flour. Then add three fourths of a tea spoonful of super carbonate of soda. Mix the whole with sweet milk and bake immediately.

To Cure Warts

Aqua Ammoniac[99], Tincture Cantharides[100] aa[101] if mix, if not the warts should be wet frequently with one of them and the other alternately every day.

Soft Gingerbread

One and a half ℔ [pounds] of flour, 12 oz of sugar, 8 eggs. Ginger to your taste, pearlash[102].

Cookies

Take 3 ℔ [pounds] of flour, 12 oz of sugar, ½ ℔ [pounds] of butter ½ pint milk, 2 teaspoonfuls pearlash.

French Loaf

1 ℔ [pound] of sugar, 1 ℔ [pound] of flour, ½ ℔ [pound] butter, ½ a ℔ [pound]

---

99 Ammonium Hydroxide.
100 A preparation made from blister beetles, a poison. Also called tincture of Spanish flies.
101 equal parts
102 Potassium carbonate

raisins & Eggs half a Lemon nutmeg

Imitation Oysters

Take young green corn & grate it in a dish
to 1 pt of this add 1 egg well beaten a small
tea cup full of flour half a cup of Butter
some salt & pepper & mix them well together
a table spoonfull of these will make the size
of an Oyster fry them a little brown and
when done butter them. Cream if it can
be procured is better than Butter

To Clean Gloves

Cream of Tartar rubbed upon soiled
white kid Gloves will cleanse them

Good Custard

boil a pt of milk with Lemon peel
& a stick of cinnamon. when it is
boiling beat up the yelk of 5 Eggs
with a pt of Cream. when the milk
tastes of the spice pour it into the

raisins, 8 eggs, half a lemon, nutmeg.

Imitation Oysters

Take young green corn and grate it in a dish. To 1 pint of this add 1 egg well beaten, a small tea cup full of flour, half a cup of butter, some salt and pepper, and mix them well together.
A table spoonful of these will make the size of an oyster. Fry them a little brown and when done, butter them. Cream, if it can be measured, is better than butter.

To Clean Gloves

Cream of tartar rubbed upon soiled whited gloves will cleanse them.

Good Custard

Boil a pint of milk with lemon peel and a stick of cinnamon. When it is boiling beat up the yolk of 5 eggs with a pint of cream. When the milk tastes of the spices pour into the

Cream stirring well then sweeten as you like it. Give the custard a simmer till a proper thickness but not let it boil (stir one way) season with a little rose water or any thing you like put into cups & grate on nutmeg

To clean Bed ticks
Apply polend starch by rubbing it on thick with a wet cloth place it in the sun. when dry rub it with the hands. Repeat it if necessary the soiled part will be as clean as new

To make a soiled Coat look as good as new first clean the coat from Grease & dirt. Then take one gal strong decoction of logwood made by Boyling logwood chips in water. Strain this liquid & when cool add 2 oz of Gum arabic in powder which should be kept in well stopped bottles for use. Then go gently over the coat with a sponge wet

cream stirring well, then sweeten as you like it. Give the custard a simmer till a proper thickness but not let it boil (stir one way). Season with a little rose water or anything you like, put into cups and grate on the nutmeg.

To Clean Bed Ticks

Apply Poland Starch[103] by rubbing it in thick with a wet cloth, place it in the sun. When dry, rub it with the hands. Repeat it if necessary, the soiled part will be clean as new.

To make a soiled Coat look as good as new

First, clean the coat from grease and dirt, then take one gal strong decoction of dogwood made by boiling dogwood chips in water. Strain this liquid and when cool add 2 oz of gum Arabic in powder which should be put in well stopped bottles for use. Then go gently over the coat with a sponge wet

---

103 Potato starch

in the above liquid diluted to suit the colour & hang in the shade to dry. After which brush the nap smooth & it will look as good as new. The liquid will suit all brown or dark colours if properly diluted if which it is easy to judge

To Extract Grease Spot

Grease of the very worst kind (whale oil for instance) may be extracted eaven from silks ribbons and other delicate articles by means of Camphine Oil. As this oil is the better for being fresh, get but little at a time. Pour some camphine in to a cup & dip lightly with a clean soft white rag with this rub the grease spot. Then take take a fresh rag dipt in the camphine & continue rubbing till the grease is extracted which will be very soon. The colour of the article will be uninjured. To remove the Turpentine Odor of the camphine rub the place with cologne water or strong spirits

in the above liquid diluted to suit the colour and hang in the shade to dry. After which brush the nap smooth. It will look as good as new. The liquid will suit all brown or dark colours if properly diluted if which it is easy to judge.

To Extract Grease Spots

Grease of the very worst kind (whale oil for instance) may be extracted even from silks, ribbons, and other delicate articles by means of camphine oil.[104] As this oil is the better for being fresh, get but little at a time. Pour some camphine in 60 a cup & dip lightly with a clean, soft, white rag. With this rub the grease spot. Then take a fresh rag dipped in the camphine and continue rubbing till the grease is extracted which will be very soon. The colour of the article will be uninjured. To remove the turpentine odor of the camphine, rube the place with cologne water or strong spirits

---

104 Camphine was the trade name of a purified spirit of turpentine formerly used for lamps, generally prepared by distilling turpentine with quicklime.

of wine & expose it to the open air repeat this process if any oder remains after the first

To make Sweet Cider
Put in a tub 5 gallons Luke warm water. put in the water 30 tb common brown sugar (6 or 7 cents) also 1 tb 2oz Tartaric acid & three pints Brewers yeast all well disolved put them in a barrel, then put in 25 gal more of water (cold) let it stand to work off the yeast with the bung out; when worked put in the bung ready)

To make Japan Liquid Blacking
1 pint spirits wine
3 oz Venice Turpentine
2 Tablespoonfulls of ivory black
1½ oz Gum shillac
all put in together stand 48 hours fit for use

of wine and expose it to the open air. Repeat this process if any odor remains after the first.

To Make Sweet Cider

Put in a tub 5 gallons lukewarm water. Put in the water 30 ℔s [pounds] common brown sugar (6 or 7 cents) also 1 ℔ [pound] 2 oz tartaric acid and three pints brewer's yeast all well dissolved. Put them in a barrel then put in 25 gal more of water (cold). Let it stand to work off the yeast with the bung[105] out. When worked, put in the bung neatly

To make Japan Liquid Blacking

1 pint spirits wine
3 oz Venice turpentine
2 table spoonfuls of ivory black
1½ oz gum shellac
all put in together, stand 48 hours, fit for use

---

105 The "bung" is the tap of the cask

Mead

To make mead a wholesome & plesant drink
- 2 quarts water
- 2   "   Molasses
- 5   oz Tartaric Acid
- 5   "   Winter Green Essence
- 1   "   Lemon
- 1   "   Soff of Sas

all mixed together then take the white of 2 Eggs & beat up in spirits & Brown sugar & add to the above syrup. Take 2 Tablespoonfulls of the syrup to a glass ⅔ Pint full of water foam with Soda

To make Cream Nectar

Take 12 tts of Sugar 12 oz Tartaric Aci 3 quarts water put them in a clean brass Kettle on the fire when warm add the white of 12 Eggs & 12 Tablespoonfulls of wheat flour beat up well together to the above. When it cools 3 minutes take it off & put it in a Keg to cool when cold add 3 gills of any Kind of Essence to the

Mead

To make Mead, a wholesome and pleasant drink.
2 quarts water
2 quarts molasses
5 oz Tartaric Acid
5 oz Wintergreen Essence
1 oz Lemon
1 oz Sassafras
All mixed together, then take the white of 2 eggs and beat up in spirits and brown sugar and add to the above syrup. Take 2 tablespoonfuls of the syrup to a pint glass 2/3 full of water, foam with soda.

To Make Cream Nectar

Take 12 lbs [pounds] of sugar, 12 oz tartaric acid, 3 quarts water, put them in a clean brass kettle on the fire. When warm add the white of 12 eggs and 12 tablespoonfuls of wheat flour. Beat up well together to the above. When it cools 3 minutes, take it off and put it in a jug to cool. When cold, add 3 gills of any kind of essence to the

Above quantity, (directions for use)
Take 2 Tablespoonfulls of Nectar to a
little super Carbonate of soda to each
glass the rest water

(To make good vinegar)
Boil slowly for one hour 3 lbs coarse
Brown sugar in 3 gallons water when
cool add ½ pt yeast put it in a
cask paste a piece a piece of
Brown paper over the Bung hole
expose to the Sun or warm place
in the house (Good in 8 or 10 days
& Good for pickels)

Howels Washing Solution
Take of Camphine &
Spts of Turpentine eaqual
parts and to one quart of this
solution add two oz of hartshorn
well pulverised and mix them well
Together
Directions for useing

above quantity (directions for use)
Take a tablespoonful of nectar to a little sugar, carbonate of soda to each glass, the rest water.

(To make good vinegar)

Boil slowly for one hour 3 ℔s [pounds] coarse brown sugar in 3 gallons water. When cool add ½ pint yeast, put it in a cask, paste a piece of brown paper over the bung[106] hose, expose to the sun or warm place in the house. (Good in 8 or 10 days and good for pickles).

Housel's Washing Solution

Take of camphine[107] and spirits of turpentine equal parts and to one quart of this solution add two oz of hartshorn[108], well pulverized and mix them well together.
Directions for using:

---

106 A "bung" is the tap of the cask.
107 Camphine was the trade name for a purified spirit of turpentine formerly used for lamps, generally prepared by distilling turpentine with quicklime.
108 aqueous ammonia solution used as smelling salts, formerly prepared from the horns of deer.

Mix four Tablespoons full of this composition with one quart of soap, or three Tablespoonsfull with one lb of bar Soap. Then soap the clothes, with the warm suds, and put them in, let them stand 20 minutes; then soap them again; and put them in cold water, in which they are to stay 15 minutes; then boil in the same water, after which they must be sudsed and rinsed. Care should be taken to have them rinsed clean.

    The best now in use
Patented July 7 1848 (sic Gratia)

Medicated Indian   Oil

Linseed oil 1 pint Spts turpentine 1 pint Oil vitriol 1 oz, mix the oil and turpentine by shaking well in a stone jug; next you will slowly drop in the oil vitriol, by little and little, and shake the jug every half minute until the vitriol is all mixed & not leave shaking the jug til the medicine is cool, if you

Mix four tablespoons full of this composition with one quart of soap, or three tablespoons full, with one ℔ [pound] of the bar soap. Then soap the clothes, make warm suds, and put them in. Let them stand 20 minutes; then soap them again; and put them in cold water, in which they are to stay 15 minutes Then boil in the same water, after which they must be sudsed and rinsed. Care should be taken to have them rinsed clean. The best now in use. Patented July 7, 1848 (Dii Gratia)

Medicated Indian Oil

Linseed oil 1 pint, spirits turpentine 1 pint, oil vitriol 1 oz. Mix the oil and turpentine by shaking well in a stone jug; next you will slowly drop in the oil vitriol by littles and littles and shake the jug every half minute until the vitriol is all mixed and not leave shaking the jug till the medicine is cool, if you

38 use a glass vessel to prepare it in you must a very strong bottle, this med is unrivaled for the following complaints, (viz) pain in the joints & else where Cramps in the limbs burns, Scalds, frozen limbs, Chillanes, rheumatism pains in the back or side cold or ague in the face and breast, neuralgia, tic doloreaux, nervous pains, tooth ache, Sciatica, bruises, Sprains, strains, fresh cuts or wounds, old sores of every desercption gangrenous ulcerates ill conditioned sore legs &c. for hors flesh there is not a medicen more applicable. for windgalls, Sodells, galds, pole evil, sweenea, fistula's corking near the huff cuts bruises &c &c — it remoues the pain & smarting of burnes in five minuits

A sure cure for stifle in Horses
Take one Gal urine & put therein a small handfull of Plug Tobacco boil down to one quart then add two ounces oil spice 1 oz al Amber two spoonfulls of spts Turpentine & 2 do of honey. put it in a Jug and cork it tight for use, process of application rub the stifle bone hard with meture 15 or 20 minutes then dry it in thronoughly with a red hot shovel. then ride the horse forth and back 100 yds. Repeat the above 2 or 3 times and the cure will be affected

use a glass vessel to prepare it in, you must use a very strong bottle. This med is unrivaled for the following complaints (biz) pain the joints and elsewhere, cramps in the limbs, burns, scalds, frozen limbs, chilblains, rheumatism, pains in the back or side, cold or ague in the face and breast, neuralgia, tic douloureux, nervous pains, toothache, sciatica, bruises, sprains, fresh cuts or wounds, old sores of every descriptions, gangrenous ulcerative, if conditioned sore legs for hare flesh, there is not a medicine more applicable. For wind galls, saddle galls, poll evil, sweeney, fistula's corking, near the half cuts, bruises. It remains, the pain and smarting of burns in five minutes.

Sure Cure for Stifle in Horses

Take one gal urine and put therein a small handful of ??? tobacco. Boil down to one quart, then add two ounces oil spice, 1 oz of amber, two spoonfuls of spirits turpentine and 2 do of honey. Put it in a jug and cork it tight for use. Process of application: rub the stifle bone hard with mixture 15 or 20 minutes, then dry it in thoroughly with a red hot shovel. Then ride the horse forth and back 100 yds. Repeat the above 2 or 3 times and the cure will be affected.

To take Mildew out of linnen

Rub it well with hard Soap then scrape some of into chalk & rub that also in the linnen, let it lie on the grass; as it dries, wet it a little more, and the mildew will come out.

To set fast Colours in calico & other goods — dissolve one tablespoonfull of gall in a gallon of warm water, & wash the article in it without Soap

To perfume clothes & prevent moths
Take cloves, ceder, & Rhubarb, ach one oz; pulverize & sprinkle it the chest or drawer

Cheap Paint
Take 6 tts of Melted Pitch, one pt of Linced oil, & one tb of yellow ochre. (for rough wood)

To Cure hams
Rock salt 7 tb, Saltpetre 6 oz, Molapes 3 pts, for 110 tb of meat

To take Mildew out of Linen

Rub it well with hard soap, then scrape some fine chalk and rub that also in the linen, let it lie on the grass; as it dries, wet it a little more, and the mildew will come out.

To set fast Colours in Calico and other Goods

Dissolve one tablespoonful of gall in a gallon of warm water and wash the article in it without soap.

To perfume clothes and prevent moths

Take cloves, cedar and rhubarb, each one oz, pulverize and sprinkle it in the chest or drawer.

Cheap Paint

Take 6 ℔s [pounds] of melted pitch, one pint of linseed oil and one ℔ [pound] of yellow ochre (for rough wood)

To Cure Hams

Rock salt 9 ℔s [pounds], saltpeter 6 oz, molasses 3 pints, for 100 ℔s [pounds] of meat

Water Proof for Leather.

Linseed Oil 1 pt; yellow wax, white
terpentine, each 2 oz; Burgundy pitch, 1 oz.
melt & colour with lamp Black

Valuable Eye water
Sulphate of Zink   10 gr.
Sugar Lead   20 "
Rose water   1 pt.

Disolve each seperately, then mix &
filter through blotting paper

Chil Blains
A certain cure is to have the hands or
feet or whenever the Itching is felt well
rubbed with snow & then dried. do
this morning & night for 3 days & all will be right

To banish Mosquitoes
Sprinkle a little Broon sugar on
some hot coals in your room it will
certainly banish them for the night

Water Proof for Leather

Linseed Oil 1 pint; yellow wax, white turpentine each 2 oz; Burgundy pitch 10 ℥ [℥=ounce]. Melt and colour with lamp black.

Valuable Eye Water

Sulphate of Zinc 10 grain
Sugar Lead[109] 20 grain
Rose Water 1 pint
Dissolve each separately then mix and filter through blotting paper.

Chilblains

A certain cure is to have the hands or feet or wherever the itching is felt well rubbed with snow and then dried. Do this morning and night for 3 days and all will be right.

To banish Mosquitoes

Sprinkle a little brown sugar on some hot coals in your room; it will certainly banish them for the night.

---

109 Lead acetate, a poison

How to cut an acquaintance

if he is poor lend him some money
if he is rich ask him to lend you some
    both means are certain

Brandy Rect

Take proof Spirit or good whisky
one pt add one oz Best Brandy & 30 drops
Sulphuric Acid. before adding your brandy
& acid, stain with red Sanders or logwood —
to the right colour

Adhesive Plaster

Rosin 7 parts Mutton Tallow 6 parts
melt the Rosin and tallow and
stir in sol: ammonia boil a little
and while hot pour of all but
the dreggs into cold watter and
work it the same as wax

Cough med.

Ext of Liquirice ʒi simmer in hot Gum
Arabic ʒii watter till dissolved Paragoric
Antimonial wine ʒi Dose from a tea to
a table spoonfull

How to cut an acquaintance

If he is poor, lend him some money.
If he is rich, ask him to lend you some.
Both means are certain.

Brandy Red[110]

Take proof spirit or good whiskey one pint, add one oz best brandy and 30 drops sulfuric acid. Before adding your brandy and acid, line with Red Saunders[111] or logwood[112] to the right color.

Adhesive Plaster

Rosin 11 parts, mutton tallow[113] 6 parts, melt the rosin and tallow and stir in dole ammonia. Boil a little and a while hot pour of all but the dregs into cold water and work it the same as wax.

Cough Med

Ext of licorice ʒI [ʒ=ounce] simmer in hot gum Arabic ʒii water till dissolved. Paregoric[114], Antimonial wine[115] ʒii. Dose from a tea to a table spoonful.

---

110 A dye
111 Santalinus, or Red Sandalwood
112 It is the blood-red heartwood that is used for dyeing.
113 Rendered fat from cattle or sheep
114 camphorated tincture of opium
115 Antimony and potassium tartarate

Eye Water

One quart Rain or distilled water one quart of pure cider vinegar or white wine vinegar white vitriol ½ oz Salt rebrained in or over the fire ¼ oz mix & reduce as may be needed to fit the eyes openly it to the out side and on the inside of the eye use laxitive med before and at the time of using the med

For the Croup

Take a part of hornets nest and pour on boiling water sweeten it with honey or sugar give a tea spoonful or a table spoon full it will not make them sick nor hurt them

Staining guns

1 and ½ oz of tincture of steel ½ oz of corrosive sublimate 1½ oz of Spirits nitre 1 oz blue vitriol ¾ oz of nitric acid or aquafortis to be added to one quart soft water & one & a ½ oz spirits wine

Eye Matter

One quart rain or distilled water. One quart of pure cider vinegar or white wine vinegar, white vitriol[116] ½ oz. Sault browned on or over the fire ½ oz, mix. A reduce as may be needed to fit the eyes openly it to the outside and on the inside of the eye use laxative med before and at the time of using the med.

For the Croup

Take a part of hornet's nest and pour on boiling water, sweeten it with honey or sugar, give a tea spoonful or a table spoonful. It will not make them sick nor hurt them.

Staining guns

Sand ½ oz of tincture of steel[117], ½ oz of corrosive sublimate[118], 1½ oz of spirits niter[119], 1 oz blue vitriol[120] ¾ oz of nitric acid or aqua fortis[121] to be added to one quart soft water pour a ½ oz spirits wine.

---

116 Zinc sulphate
117 Iron chloride
118 Mercuric chloride
119 Ethyl nitrite
120 Copper sulphate
121 Another name for nitric acid

For the Croup By B H Hale

Equal parts tincture of Bloodroot and Tincture of Lobelia Dose one teaspoonful every 5 minutes soke the feet in warm water and wring cloths in hot water and lay them on the chest and bowels

Dropsy by B H Hale

Podophilin ¼ grn with half tea spoonful Cream Tarter every 2 hours until it produces half dozen copious discharges from the bowels and repeat in 2 or 3 days afterwards to produce the same effects in any kind of dropsy.

Green Salve

Lard ½ pound Beeswax 2 oz white turpentine ¼ pound Rosin 2 oz pure honey 2 oz melt all slowly and compactly together when part cool add 1 and ½ oz pulverized verdigris stir well and let settle and pour off the clean part from the verdigris make into rolls for use of ____ sore old sores fresh cuts and wounds on man or beast

For the Croup By B. F. Hale

Equal parts tincture of bloodroot and tincture of lobelia. Dose: one teaspoonful every 5 minutes, soak the feet in warm water and wring cloths in hot water and lay them on the chest and bowels.

Dropsy by B. F. Hale

Podophyllin[122] ½ grain with half teaspoonful cream tartar every 2 hours until it produces half dozen copious discharges from the bowel and repeat in 2 or 3 days. Afterwards to produce the same effects in any kind of dropsy.

Gum Salve

Lard ½ pound, Beeswax 2 oz, white turpentine ½ pound, rosin 2 oz, pure honey 2 oz, melt aa slowly and compactly together, when partly cooled add lard ½ oz pulverized verdigris[123]. Stir well and let settle and pour off the clean part from the verdigris. Make into pills for sale. Use for scrofulous sores, all old sores, first cuts and wounds on man or beast.

---

122 Podophyllum Resin is the powdered mixture of resins removed from the May apple or Mandrake
123 Copper carbonate

44 X Mothers, Stomach bitters or Cordial, very good in all debility of the Stomach aids digestion, appetite & general debility —
Take Gentian root ground 1 & 1/2 oz, Orange peal 2 & 1/2 oz, Cinnamon 1/4 oz, anise seed 1/2 oz, Coriander Seed 1/2 oz, unground peruvian bark 1/2 oz, Gum kino 1/4 oz, pound all moderately fine & add one quart alcohol let stand 2 weeks, shaking occasionally, pour off the clear tincture & put in it one pound Crushed or loaf Sugar & 4 quarts Clear water, it can be pouned off or it may stan on the dregs,,, I pass it through the perculator & bring it very clear, but not essential — A good medicine

X
My bathing drops, Good Alcohol one quart, or liniment, & add oil Sassafras, oil hemlock,
X spts turpentine each 1/2 an oz, Chloroform 3/4 oz, tinc Catachu, tinc Goac each 1/2 oz, Oil origanum 1 oz, Oil Wintergreen 2 drachms & 1/8 oz, Gum Camp 2 drachms, mix all together shake well & it is fit for use, for pains in any part the body, like rheumatism neuralgia &c, & to be taken for pain in stomach & bowels. N.B. add tinc Myrrh 2 oz tinc Cayenne 1/2 oz, Laudanum 1/2 oz = good

Mathers Stomach Bitters or Cordial

Very good in all debility of the stomach. Aids in digestion, appetite, and general debility. Take gentian root[124] ground 1½ oz, orange peel 2½ oz, cinnamon ¼ oz, anise seed ½ oz, coriander seed, ½ oz, unground Peruvian bark[125] ½ oz, gum Kino[126] ¼ oz, pound all moderately fine and add one quart alcohol. Let stand 2 weeks, shaking occassionally. Pour off the clean tincture spirit in it. One pound crushed or loaf sugar and 4 quarts of clear water, it can be poured off or it may stan on the dregs. I pass it through the percolator and bring it very clear but not essential. A good medicine.

My Bathing Drops

Good alcohol one quart, or liniment and add oil sassafras, oil hemlock, spirits turpentine, each ½ oz, chloroform ¾ oz, tincture catechu[127], tincture Gouch[128], each ½ oz, oil Origanum[129] 1 oz, oil wintergreen, 2 drachms and 1/8 oz, gum camp(hor) 2 drachms, mix all together, shake well and it is fit for use, for pains in any part of the body like rheumatism, neuralgia. To be taken for pain in stomach and bowels, N.b. Add tinc Myrrh 2 grain, tinc cayenne ½ oz, laudanum[130] ½ oz. Good.

---

124 Gentian is an herb.
125 Jesuit's bark, also known as cinchona bark, Peruvian bark, or China bark, is a former name of a supposed remedy for malaria, as the bark contains quinine used to treat the disease.
126 Kino is a botanical gum
127 extract of acacia trees
128 a potent blend of antioxidants and herbs
129 Thymus capitatus
130 tincture of opium

Phloridzine ⅔ Wild Cherry bark 2 oz 45
to make   Liquirice root 1 oz, 4 drachms
If On big Bark Blood root ½ oz 4 drachms
I have got   Black Cohosh ½ oz 4 drachms
this, Wallace Red Saunders ½ oz, 1 drachm,
pound all moderately fine put in one pint
hot water let stand 48 hours & add one
pint Alcohol let stand from one day to
14 & add 4 oz Crushed Sugar, disolve,
& let stand 24 hours, strain, add
tinc Ipicac 3 oz, tinc Lobelia 3 drachms,
wine of antimony 3 oz, Laudanum 3 drachms
Irun the tinc through the dregs a number
times to make it clear in the percalater
but it will do without letting it stand
& pour off the clear part from the sediment.

To remove pimpels from the face
Alumn one ounce
Borax " ⅓ "
pound them fine and desolve
in water either soft or hard
then apply to the face by
means of fine colth let the
water dry on the face.

Phlorizin[131]—to make
(on big book[132], I got this—Wallace)

Wild cherry bark 2 oz, licorice root ½ oz 4 drachms, bloodroot ½ oz 4 drachms, black cohosh ½ oz 4 drachms, Red Saunders 1/8 oz 1 drachm. Pound all moderately fine. Put in one pint hot water. Let stand 48 hours and add 1 pint alcohol. Let stand from one day to 14 and add 4 oz crushed sugar, dissolve. Let stand 24 hours, strain, add tinc Ipecac 2 oz, tinc lobelia 2 drachms, wine of antimony[133] 3 oz, laudanum 3 drachms. I run the tinc through the dregs a number of times to make it clear in the percolator, but it will do without; letting it stand and pour off the clear part from the sediment.

To Remove Pimples from the Face

Alum one ounce
Borax one 1/3 ounce
Pound them fine and dissolve in water either soft or hard then apply to the face by means of a fine cloth. Let the matter dry on the face.

---

131 glycoside of phloretin
132 Lois Hale Reid has this big book
133 Antimony and Potassium tartrate

Dr Hales best Linement

Linseed oil one quart
Hemlock oil   4 oz
Red or White Cedar oil   4 oz
Organum oil   4 oz
oil Spike   4 oz
Rectified oil Amber   4 oz
Gum Opium   2 oz
Gum Camphor   2 oz
Niter   2 oz
Spts Amenia   1 lb
"   Turpentine   1 Pt
Alcohol   1 Pt

Desolve the oils in the Alcohol and Mix

Eye Watter

Take sulphate of zink one part
Crocus Martus two parts
put into rain watter two qts

Dr. Hale's Best Liniment

Linseed oil one quart
Hemlock oil 4 oz
Red or White Cedar oil 4 oz
Origanum oil 4 oz
Oil Spike[134] 4 oz
Rectified oil amber 4 oz
Gum Opium 2 oz
Gum Camphor 2 oz
Niter 2 oz
Spirits Ammonia 1 lb
Spirits Turpentine 1 pint
Alcohol 1 pint
Dissolve the oils in the alcohol and mix

Eye Matter

Take sulfate of zinc one part, Crocus Martis[135] two parts, put in rain water two quarts.

---

134 Lavender Spike Oil
135 Spanish red iron oxide

Tooth Ache

Solution of carbonate of Amonia & any commentine to be held in the mouth and put in the tooth

July 12 = 62
For ringworm — Simple Cerate, with a very little corrocive Sublimate & a little acitate zinc mix under a knife perfectly & use prudently —

My best Linament — Alcohol 1 quart ״ oil sasafras 4 oz ״ oil hemlock 2 oz ״ Spts turpentine 5 oz ״ Chloroform 4 oz ״ tincture goacl 2 oz ״ oil origanum 1 oz ״ oil wintergreen 2 drachms Gum Camph 2 drachms, tinc Myrrh 2 oz ״ tinc Cayenne 4 oz ״ Laudanum 2 oz ״ tinc of red sounders enough to give the colour desired

For Neuralgia & — take my bathing drops 1 oz ״
pain in the head — aqua Ammonia 2 drachms
Chloroform 2 drachms
Laudanum 2 drachms, and rub a little painted part often & often smaller rub about much.

Tooth Ache

Solution of carbonate of ammonia and any common tinc to be held in the mouth and put in the tooth.

July 12 = 62 For Ringworm

Simple Cerate[136], with a very little corrosive sublimate[137] and a little acetate zinc[138], mix under a knife perfectly and use prudently.

My Best Liniment

Alcohol 1 quart, oil sassafras ½ oz, oil hemlock ½ oz, spirits turpentine 2 oz, chloroform ¾ oz, tinc Gouch ½ oz, oil Origanum 1 oz, oil wintergreen 2 drachms, gum camphor 2 drachms, tinc myrrh 2 oz, tinc cayenne ½ oz, laudanum ½ oz, tinc of Red Saunders, enough to give the colour desired.

For Neuralgia and Pain in the Head

Take my bathing drops 1 oz, aqua ammonia 2 drachms, chloroform 2 drachms, laudanum 2 drachms, mix and for the pained par often and often smell or inhale, as much

---

136 a mixture of three parts of paraffin and seven parts of lard
137 Mercuric chloride
138 a salt with the formula $Zn(CH_3CO_2)_2$

as cancer eases, brown & that subject is hand
you will wet a cloth & apply to the parts &
do it often wetting it, keep it applied
for a good length of time.

Cancer Plaster & Arsenic, Rochell Salts,
White vitriol, Sulphur, aqua
fortis, mixed with the yelk of egg, to the
consistency of batter or flapjacks before being
baked & bake in an oven or stove til
done or til it rises up, put all in a
clean new earthen dish
add to the above a little or ¾ part of Corrosive Sublimate
or ¼ fourth [or] it as much as there is of
any one of the other articles.

To the plaster add the yelk of egg & apply it spread
on cloth of cotton or silk; change the plaster every
day or two until the cancer looks black & begins
to turn [?] a little round the edges then you
will apply a poultice of slippery elm or bread
& milk, after 24 or 36 hours, apply the cancer
plaster again, & continually till cancer is killed
& then apply the simple Cerate to heal it.

as can be easily borne. If neuralgia is hard you will wet a cloth and apply to the pained part often wetting it. Keep it applied for a good length of time.

Cancer Plaster

Essence Rochelle Salts[139], white vitriol[140], sulfur, equal parts mixed with the yolk of egg, to the consistency of batter of flapjacks before being baked and bake in an oven or stove till done or till it rises up, put all in a clean new earthen dish.

Add to the above a little or ¼ part of corrosive sublimate[141] and ¼ or fourth part as much as there is of any of the other articles.

Mix the plaster with the yolk of eggs and apply it spread on cloth of cotton or silk. Change the plaster every day or two until the cancer looks black and begins to discharge a little around the edges, then you will apply a poultice of slippery elm or bread and milk. After 24 or 36 hours, apply the cancer plaster again, so continue the cancer is killed. Apply simple cerate[142] to heal it.

---

139 Potassium sodium tartrate
140 Zinc sulfate
141 Mercuric chloride
142 How to make: page 70

X ~~for pain in stomach, bowels, Diarrhea,~~
~~Cholera morbus, spasms, like in Colic, & for~~
~~external use, with nervous pains~~
~~Compound Spts Lavender~~
~~Sulphuric Ether~~
~~Tincture of Cayenne~~
~~Ess ginger~~
~~Laudanum   drachm~~
~~may & take from 10 drops to a teaspoonful in~~
~~cold weak tea or sweetened water~~

Diptheria } Strong Sage tea   ½ pint
              Salt 2 table spoonfuls
         X   honey strained 2 table spoonfuls
              Vinegar best 2 table spoonfuls
              Cayenne one tea spoonful mix
take a little often & gargle the throat
every hour freely

Rheumatic Liniament } 1 Pt Alcohol
add 4 oz Beefs gall let stand 48 hours
then add 4 oz Spts Hartshorn next add 1
oz Oil Sassafras 1 oz oil Lavender you can
color it with any color you please.
        Gurd. Se says   B F Hall, M H Ruttan

For pain in stomach, bowels, diarrhea, cholera morbus, spasm, colic and for external use with nervous pains
Compound spirits lavender 2 oz
Sulfuric ether[143] 1 oz
Tincture of Cayenne 1 oz
Tinc ginger 2 oz
Laudanum drachm 2
Mix and take from 20 drops to one teaspoonful in cold weak tea or sweet water.

Diphtheria

Strong sage tea ½ pint
Salt 2 table spoonfuls
honey, strained 2 table spoonfuls
Vinegar best 2 table spoonfuls
Cayenne one teaspoonful mix.
Take a little often and gargle the throat every hour freely.

Rheumatic Liniment

1 pint alcohol, add 4 oz Beefs gall. Let stand 48 hours then add spirits hartshorn next, add 1 oz oil sassafras, 1 oz oil lavender. You can color the urine any color you please.
Good, so says B. F. Hale, M. L. Ruttance

---

[143] Diethyl ether

50
Itch Ointment) One plug tobacco, handfull Catnip
x 5 Tea Spoonfull pepper do Ginger do Salt 2 teasp-
oonfulls Sulpher. One lb Butter or lard with a
little mutton tallow. boil the Catnip & tobacco in
sperits and watter to git all the stregnth. Simmer
in the lard untill the Watter disaperes then add
the other articles pulverized.

Cement for uniting) Equal parts of Pitch. Rosin
   my Cupping glasses) and Beeswax with a little

Fit drops for x) Gum Myrr ʒj Sulpher ʒj
Epilepsy (Infalible.) Olive oil one gill Spts Turpentine half pt the Sulpher Myrrh and oil must be
mixed and melted together and boil or stir untill
red then add the turpentine after it is removed
from the fire. Dose. From 2 to 25 drops, once
or twice a day in a little Brandy or wine to
be continued but first cleanse the Stomach
with Emitec or Physic,

Healing Salve) Rosin & Beeswax each 1 lb
Mutton tallow ʒij Gum Camphor ʒj tinc
Myrrh — ʒj melt the rosin beeswax and tallow
then add the Myrrh tinc & Camphor finely
powered when all are melted strain through a

Itch Ointment

One plug tobacco handful, catnip teaspoonful, pepper do, ginger do, salt 2 teaspoonfuls, sulfur one lb, Butter or lard with a little mutton tallow. Boil the catnip and tobacco in spirits and water to get all the strength. Simmer in the lard until the water disappears, then add the other articles pulverized.

Cement for Uniting My Cupping Glasses

Equal parts of pitch, rosin, and beeswax with a little...

Fit drops for Epilepsy, Infallible

Gum myrrh ℨj [ℨ=ounce], Sulfur ℨj, olive oil one gill, spirits turpentine half pint. The sulfur, myrrh and oil must be mixed and melted together, and boil or stir until red then add the turpentine after it is removed from the fire. Dose: From 2 to 25 drops once or twice a day in a little Brandy or wine to be continued but first cleanse the stomach with emetic or physic.

Healing Salve

Rosin and beeswax each 1 lb, mutton tallow ℨij [ℨ=ounce], Gum Camphor ℨj, tinc myrrh ℨj. Melt the rosin, beeswax, and tallow, then add the myrrh, tinc and camphor finely powered when all are melted. Strain through a

fine cloth return to the kettle add the tinct
Myrrh when all are well incorporated pour
the mass into Watter and work it like wax,
this is usefull as a strenghening plaster and
a salve for ulcers of every discription haveing been used with the most astonishing success. BH
Worms) Bitter root is the best above all
    be sure and try it.
Blue Cohush it's properties (ammung the deascases and uses   in which it is usefull
is Colic Cholera morbus, Epilepsy, Hustericus
and every other spicies of fits Feven ague – Inflamation
of the Uterius and for Worms good to unite with
cathartics to prevent it's griping a powerful antispozmetic in any case and perfectly safe.
(Lucy's ague) Put in three half pts of good Brandy
  Bitters ×) or other good spirits one oz Golden
  Seal pulverised half oz good Composition half
  oz Bloodroot. Doce all the Stomache will
bear 3 or 4 times a day B.H. Hale.
Caugh Balsam) Fir Balsam 2 oz honey 2 oz
alcohol 1 pt let stand closely corked 10 days
shaking it often then filter and add 3 gills

fine cloth, return to the kettle, add the tinct myrrh when all are well evaporated. Pour the mass into water and work it like wax. This is useful as a strengthening plaster and a salve for ulcers of every description, having been used with the most astonishing success. B.F.

Worms

Bitterroot is the best above all, be sure and try it.

Blue Cohosh—its properties and uses

Among the diseases in which it is useful is Colic, Cholera Morbus, Epilepsy, Hysterics, and every other species of fits, and even ague. Inflammation of the Uterus and for Worms. Good to unite with cathartics[144] to prevent its gripping. A powerful antispasmodic[145] in any case and perfectly safe.

Lucy's Ague

Put in three half-pints of good Brandy, Bitters x or other good spirits one oz Golden Seal pulverized, half oz good Composition, half oz bloodroot. Dose: all the stomach will bear 3 or 4 times a day. B. F. Hale

Cough Balsam

Fir Balsam 2 oz, honey 2 oz, alcohol 1 pint. Let stand closely corked 10 days shaking it often then filter and add 3 gills

---

144 Purgative drugs
145 used to relieve spasm of involuntary muscle.

tincture Leobelia., Dose from one half to a teaspoonful several times a day good for Coughs, Asthma pain in the Breast, Croup, gravel, dropsy, ghonorrhoea, Nerve and Bone)

X Linneament (Oil organum 1 lb Oil Rosemary 1 lb Olive Oil 2 lbs tinct cantharides ½ lb Sperits turpentine ½ pd Strangert xpts Camphor 1 oz mix all well, for Scrofula inflamation, Chronic rheumatism, Wounds on man or beast scalds spiains, Bruses., Contraction of cords and sinews and even to bathe the palpebra muscles of the eyes in case of inflaimation or sore eyes, B H 74

Cough Powders) Wild turnips ʒj Blood Root ʒjß Skunk cabbage ʒj Lobelia ʒj, Comfrey Root ʒjv Cayenne ʒjß, Leadys Slipper ʒjjj Elecampane ʒj, Opium ℈j Lof Sugar ʒjj all pulverised and well mixed) Dose from ½ to a tea spoonful for an adult and less for an under age)

tincture lobelia. Dose: from one half to a teaspoonful several times a day. Good for cough, fits, asthma, pain in the breast, croup, gravel, dropsy, gonorrhea.

Nerve and Bone Liniment

Oil origanum 1 lb, Oil Rosemary 1 lb, olive oil 2 lbs tinct cantharides ½ lb, spirits turpentine ½ pint, Strangert? spirits camphor 1 oz. Mix all well. For scrofula inflammation, chronic inflammation, wounds on man or beast, scalds, sprains, bruises, contraction of cords and sinews, and even to bathe the palpebral muscles of the eyes in case of inflammation or sore eyes. BFH

Cough Powders

Wild turnip ℨj [ℨ=ounce], Bloodroot ℨjs, Skunk Cabbage ℨj, Lobelia ℨj, Comfrey Root ℨiv Cayenne ℨ1/2, Lady's Slipper ℨiij, Elecampane[146] ℨy, Opium ℈, Loaf Sugar ℨjj. All pulverized and well mixed. Dose: from ½ to a teaspoonful for an adult and less for an underage.

---

146 Inula helenium, also called horse-heal or elfdock

x ~~Worm~~ Worm Loozenges by B H. 44

Take Apella wormseed three oz carbonate potasa one oz Slack lime sifted one half oz Watter 3½ pts put on the fire stir often with a wooden spatula let boil one half hour, take off pres through linnen cloth let settle decant add nitric acid untill it reddens litmus paper without being sensibely acid to the tounge allow it to rest pass it through a filter previously moisened or through a piece of close canvas and allow ~~the and atter~~ the product which remains on the filter, to dry in the open air untill hard as butter. For the Loozenges take three dachmes of the above powered in a marble morter add by degrees gum Arabec powered white Sugar 15 oz one and one half oz oil of lemmon 25 drops form with a sufficent quantity of watter of the right consistance form lozengers each weighing when dride 15 grains infants under 6 month the Doc is one Loozenge night and morning from 6 to one year give two from 1 to 2 years give 3 from 2 to 4

Worm Lozenges by B.F.H

Take Apella Wormseed[147], three oz carbonate potash[148], one oz slaked lime[149], sifted one half oz, water 3 ½ pints. Put on the fire, stir often with a wooden spatula, let boil one half hour. Take off, prep through linen cloth, let settle, decant, add nitric acid until it reddens litmus paper without being sensibly acid to the tongue. Allow it to rest, pass it through a filter previously moistened or through a piece of close canvas and allow the product which remains on the filter to dry in the open air until hard as butter. Take three drachms of the above in a marble mortar, add by degrees powdered white sugar 15 oz.

For the Lozenges

Preserved gum Arabic one and one half oz, oil of lemon, 25 drops. Form with a sufficient quantity of water of the right consistency form lozenges, each weighing when dried 15 grains. Infants under 6 months the dose is one lozenge night and morning. From 6 to one year give two, from 1 to 2 years, give three, from 2 to 4

---

147 Epazote, poisonous in large quantities
148 Potassium carbonate K_2CO_3
149 Calcium hydroxide

4 night and morning for those older an
extra lozenge for each year to be give night
and morning continued untill the desired
efect are produced in every instance. Good,

) Rheumatic) R Alchol 16 gallons
Linneament (Oil wormwood 2 lbs
add Discrutionary tinct of) Oorganum 3 "
flies. Gum Camphor (Oil Sasafras 1 "
Spts turpentine, oil (Casteel Soap 1¾ "
Cageput. Oil Vitriol ½ "
flies lb1 " Camphor Capsicum annuum
lb 1 turpentine lb 1 or Cayenne 1½ "
Cageput oil z Beefs gall 1½ gall
Mix & tir often for 10 days filter for use

For the lungs) Blood root Zj Digitales 1 z
Cough &c (Cherry bark 2 oz Liquree root 2 oz
Black cohush root 2 oz onion
seed 2 oz foreign valerian 2 oz
Cold spirits percolate add Sugar tinct Ipecac
2 oz Laudanum 1 oz — to the above add 1 qt
diluted Alcohol,

4 night and morning for those older, an extra lozenge for each year to be given night and morning continued until the desired effects are produced in every instance. Good.

Rheumatic Liniment	Rx Alcohol 16 gallons
Add Discretionary tinct of flies[150], gum camphor, spirits of turpentine, oil cajeput[151]. Flies 1 lb, camphor 1 lb, turpentine 1 lb, cajeput oil ʒ [ounce]	Oil Wormwood 2 lbs
	Origanum 3 lbs
	Oil Sassafras 1 lb
	Castile Soap 1 ¾ lb
	Oil Vitriol ½ lb
	Capsicum annum or Cayenne 1½ lb
	Beef gall 1½ gallon

Mix. Stir often for 10 days, filter for use.

For the Lungs

Bloodroot ʒj [ʒ=ounce], Digitalis 1 oz, Cherry bark 2 oz, licorice root 2 oz, black cohosh root 2 oz, onion seed 2 oz, foreign valerian 2 oz. Cold spirits percolate, add sugar, tinct spice 2 oz, Laudanum 1 oz, to the above add 1 quart diluted alcohol.

---

150 Cantharides, a dangerous, sometimes fatal, preparation of powdered, dried Spanish flies
151 Melaleuca Leucadendron

Cholera Med

No 6 ℥j — Spts Camphor ½ oz
Ess Pepermint ½ oz. Laudanum ½ oz
tinc Ginger 1 oz Sudorific drops ½ oz
mix.

× Grand Ague med

Hourhoun ℥j Boneset ℥j Sassafras ℥j
Willow ℥j ——— ℥ii Sugar 3 oz Brandy 2 oz
Boil the articles down to ½ pt add the sugar
when cold add the brandy — add 1 oz wandering
milkweed to the above. to the above add ℥ß
wormwood and one oz box wood bark
Wahoo 1 oz

Corns

One tea spoonful tar. one psolt-peter one
tea spoonful coarse brown sugar. warm
the whole together spread on thin leather
the size of the corn in 3 days the corn will
be drawn out.

Cholera Med

No. 6 ʒj [ʒ=ounce], spirits camphor ½ oz, essence peppermint ½ oz, Laudanum ½ oz, tinc ginger 1 oz, sudorific[152] drops ½ oz. Mix.

Grand Ague Med

Horehound ʒj [ʒ=ounce], Boneset[153] ʒj, Sassafras ʒj, Willow ʒj, ~~~ ʒii, Sugar 3 oz, Brandy 2 oz. Boil the articles down to ½ pint. Add the sugar when cold add the brandy = add 1 oz wandering milkweed to the above. To the above add ʒjs wormwood and one oz boxwood bark, Wahoo[154] 1 oz.

Corns

One tea spoonful tar, one saltpeter, one teaspoonful coarse brown sugar, warm the whole together, spread on thin leather the size of the corn. In three days the corn will be drawn out.

---

152 Sudorifics are agents that induce the body to sweat profusely. They may be pharmacologic drugs (e.g. plant-derived drugs) or herbals such as Jamaican Ginger, Boneset, Bayberry bark, Yarrow stems and leaves, Black pepper berries, Canada snake root, and Sage leaves.
153 *Eupatorium perfolatum*
154 *Euonymus Atropurureus*

No 1. Black Salve B H. H.

Linseed oil 1 pt. Olive oil ½ pt mix slowly simmer down one third while cooling add one oz red lead continue to stir untill cold. N B. The red lead must be ground in a mortar as fine as possible and sifted in slowly good for fresh cuts old sors and the greatest remidy for burns in existance said to be a good adthesive plaster and stregngthing for the big muscles this is the best Salve in existance B H. T Ha

Cologn Watter

Oil Lavender ʒij Oil Lemon ʒiʃs
Oil Bergamont ʒij Oil Rosemary ʒj
Oil Safafras ʒʃs Oil Cinnamon ʒʃs
Oil Cloves ʒij Fine musk ʒʃs
Oil Orange gts 12 Neroli gts 6
Alcohol 1 gall

No. 1 Black Salve B.F.H.

Linseed oil 1 pint, olive oil ½ pint. Mix, slowly simmer down one third while cooling, add one oz red lead, continue to stir until cold. A. B. The red lead[155] must be ground in a mortar as fine as possible and sifted in slowly. Good for fresh cuts, old sores, and the greatest remedy for burns in existence, said to be a good adhesive plaster and strengthening for big muscles. This is the best Salve in existence. B. F. Hale

Cologne Water

Oil lavender ʒij
[ʒ=ounce]
Oil Bergamot[156] iij
Oil Sassafras ss
Oil Cloves ʒj
Oil Orange quarts 12

Oil Lemon iss
Oil Rosemary j
Oil Cinnamon ss
Fine musk[157] j
Neroli[158] quarts 6

Alcohol 1 gallon

---

155 Lead Oxide, with the formula Pb3O4
156 a plant that produces a type of citrus fruit
157 a strong-smelling reddish-brown substance which is secreted by the male musk deer for scent-marking and is an important ininedient in perfumery.
158 an essential oil produced from the blossom of the bitter orange tree

Green Salve Good

R ½ pd fresh butter do Beeswax
do white pine turpentine ¼ pd Rosin
¼ pd honey melt all together when partly cold
add ½ oz pulverised verdigris stir till cold good
for all old sores, fever sores. Scrofula, an
efectual cure for psalt Rhume with a strong
decoction of Bloodroot to wash with 2 or 3 times
@ day,

× Sweet tinct Rheubarb
Root of Rheubarb in coarse pewder 2 oz
" " Licquorice bruised, Annis seed
bruised each one oz double refined sugar in
powder 2 oz Diluted Alcohol 2 ½ pounds
digest 8 days and filter through paper
good for weak Stomach, Indigestion, and
is a mild phicie

× Lucys last cough med
Raisens cut into 4 oz Elicampain root 1/3 oz
Bloodroot 1/8 oz Spiknard root ½ oz Comfry Root ¼ oz
Licquorice Root ½ oz Skunk cabage root ½ oz
boil to one qt strain add one pd good sugar I use no spirits

B H Hall

Green Salve—Good

Rx ½ pd fresh butter, do beeswax, do white pine turpentine ¼ pint rosin ¼ pd honey. Melt all together, when partly cold add ½ oz pulverized verdigris[159]. Stir till cold. Good for all old sores, fever sores, scrofula. An effectual cure for psalt-rhuma[160] with a strong decoction of bloodroot—to wash with 2 or 3 times a day.

Sweet Tinct Rhubarb

Root of Rhubarb in coarse powder 2 oz, licorice bruised, anise seed bruised, each one oz, double refined sugar in powder 2 oz, diluted alcohol 2½ pounds. Digest 8 days and filter through paper. Good for weak stomach, indigestion and is a mild physic.

Lucy's Last Cough Med

Raisins cut into 4 oz, Elecampane root 1/8 oz, bloodroot 1/8 oz, spikenard root ½ oz, Comfrey root ¼ oz, licorice root ½ oz, skunk cabbage root ½ oz. Boil to one quart, strain, add one pd good sugar. I use no spirits.

B. F. Hale

---

159 Copper carbonate
160 polymyalgia rheumatica

Hydrophobia

Tail bone of a colt pulverised. Jaw bone of a dog burnt and pulverised. Verdigris that is scraped off a copper vessel one scruple. mix well give an adult one teaspoonful. a child ½ tea spoonful — 2 hours after give ½ tea spoonful pure copper filings in 24 hours repeat the course (Pay particular notice to this) Eat nothing Greasy

Diarrhoea

If blood passes or the stools very watery add Tinct Catachu one part equil the others

{ Spts Camphor
Tinct Rheubarb
Ess Pepermint
Tinct Cayenne
Laudenum }
Each equil parts mix and give them in doses from 10 to 60 drops according to age and the urgency of the case. Good

Another { Tinct Camphor, Ess Pepermint, Paragoric if bad Tinct Catachu and if much pain Laudanum equil proportions and if the patient is of a cold phlegmatic habit add tinct capsicum proportions as above

Hydrophobia

Fals toung(?) of a colt pulverized. Jawbone of a dog burnt and pulverized. Verdigris that is scraped off a copper vessel one scruple. Mix well. Give an adult one tea spoonful: a child ½ tea spoonful. 2 hours after give ½ tea spoonful pure copper filings. In 24 hours, repeat the course. (Pay particular notice to this) Eat nothing greasy.

Diarrhea

If blood passes or the stools very watery, add Tinct Chateaux[161], one part equal to the others.
Spirits Camphor, Tinct Rhubarb, Essence Peppermint, Tinct Cayenne, Laudanum. Each equal parts mix and give them in Doses from 10 to 60 drops according to age and the urgency of the case. Good.

Another

Tinct Camphor, essence peppermint, paregoric[162] if bad, tinct chateaux and if much pain, laudanum, equal proportions and if the patient is of a cold, phlegmatic habit add tinct capsicum proportions as above

---

161 Might have been a brand name?
162 Camphorated tincture of opium

if stomach and bowels appear loaded or pressed give Rhenbarb. Saleratus. and peppermint Ep. first to move the bowels for want of pure Saleratus use Carbonate of potassa or Saltstarter wich amts to the same Good. Better, Best not for mother. Wallace Yes tis too I made a mistake,

×) Alterative for 6 Aacts little child Elder flowers 4oz Garget root 4oz Blue flag root 4oz Gooe wood 4oz Sassafras bark 4oz Mandrake root 2oz Yellow dock Root 4oz put all in a gall watter boil and pour off 2 or 3 times strain all the tea and boil down to 2 qts add Brown sugar 2 pds bring to a boil throw of the scum as it rises let cool add good spirits one pt shake well together and give from one tea spoonful to a table spoonful 4 or 5 times a day the last on going to bed   Good   B W Hall

Dr Hales   × {" Gentian root 1½ oz
Stomach bitters   Orange peel 2½ oz
or cordial   Cinnamon bark ¼ oz
Annis seed ½ oz Chery Bark 2 oz Cardamon Seed husk and all 2 drachms unground peruvian

If stomach and bowels appear loaded or pressed, give rhubarb, saleratus and peppermint essence first to move the bowels. For want of pure saleratus, use carbonate of potash or salts tartar which amounts to the same. Good. Better, Best not for mother. Wallace.
Yes, tis too, I made a mistake.

Allerative[163] for C. Hacts little child

Elder flowers 4 oz, garget root[164] 4 oz, Blue Flag root 4 oz Guaiac wood 4 oz, sassafras bark 4 oz, mandrake root 2 oz, Yellow dock root 4 oz. Put all in a gallon water, boil and pour off 2 or 3 times. Strain all the tea and boil down to 2 quarts. Add brown sugar 2 pds. Bring to a boil, throw off the scum as it rises, let cool. Add good spirits one pint, shake well together and give from one tea spoonful to a table spoonful 4 or 5 times a day, the last on going to bed. Good. B. F. Hale.

Dr. Hales Stomach Bitters or Cordial

Gentian root 1½ oz, orange peel 2½ oz, cinnamon bark ¼ oz, anise seed ½ oz, cherry bark 2 oz, cardamon seed, husk and all 2 drachms, unground Peruvian

---

163 Probably means allergy medicine
164 Pokeweed root

60

bark one oz Gum Kino ¼ oz Red Saunders 2 drachms pound moderately add one qt Alcohol let stand 36 or 48 hours or more tightly covered transfer to the perculator and run through it two or three times set by add warm watter ennough to make in all 4 qts run over and over till all is clear and at last add the Alcohol or Rum to the watter run through perculater desolve 1 pt good white sugar. Stir tell desolved run again through perculater over and over till clear press the drugs and filter through paper or double flannel and add to the first and bottle. Good By B. H. W.

D Hales Sameritan) Alcohol 1 qt
X Lineament   Oil Sapafras ½ oz
Oil Hemloc ½ oz Sperits Terpentine ½ oz
Chloriform ¾ oz Tinc Goac ½ oz
Oil Origanum 1 oz Oil Wintergreen 2 drachms
Gum Campor 2 drachms Tinct Myrrh 2 oz
Tinct Capsicum ½ oz. mix. one of the best lineaments on Earth to be used freely exturnely and taken Inernaly in case of

bark one oz, Gum Kino ¼ oz, Red Saunders 2 drachms. Pound moderately. Add one quart alcohol let stand 36 or 48 hours or more tightly covered. Transfer to the percolator and run it through two or three times set by add warm water enough to make in all 4 quarts. Run over and over till all is clear and at last add the alcohol or rum to the water, run through percolator. Dissolve 1 pd good white sugar. Stir till dissolved. Run again through percolator over and over till clear. Press the drugs and filter through paper or double flannel and add to the first and bottle. Good. By B. F. H.

Dr. Hale's Samaritan Liniment

Alcohol 1 quart, oil sassafras ½ oz, oil hemlock ½ oz, spirits turpentine ½ oz, chloroform ¾ oz tinc guaiac, oil origanum 1 oz, oil wintergreen 2 drachms, gum camphor 2 drachms, tinct myrrh 2 oz, tinct capsicum ½ oz. Mix. One of the best liniments on Earth to be used freely externally and taken internally in case of

pain in stomach. Bowels or any internal
hard pains add to the above ½ oz of the best
laudanum <u>Good</u>

×Mothers very exelent med for pain in bowels
and stomach. By B. W.t Hall
Compound spirits Lavender   2 part
Ether Sulpheric   1 "
tinc Cayenne   1 "
tinct Ginger   2 "
Spts Camphor ~~laudanum with~~   2 "
for pain in the stomach bowels,
Dose Tea Spoonful. more if needed

laudanum 2 Drachm
be sure and not
forget this
Dr Hall

Discutient   { Cicuta leavs Tobaco each
Ointment × { 2 oz. Stramonium. Yellow
dock. Garden Nightshade, each 4 oz. Bittersweet
3 oz Simmer in spirits (omitting spirits) and water to git the
strength strain and add 18 oz lard or fresh butter
bring to a propper consistence and apply
on all tumors which are indolent Cancerous
or Scirrous & where are first showing themselves
to cary them away on the breast or elswhere

pain in stomach, bowels, or any internal hard pains. Add to the above ½ oz of the best laudanum. Good.

Another very excellent medicine for pain in bowels and stomach by B. F. Hale

Compound spirits lavender 2 parts
Ether sulfuric 1 part
tinc cayenne 1 part
tinct ginger 2 parts
spirits camphor 2 parts
laudanum 2 drachms—be sure and not forget this—Dr. Hale
For pain in stomach, bowels.
Dose: tea spoonful, more if needed

Discutient Ointment

Cicuta leaves[165], tobacco each 2 oz. Stramonium[166], Yellow dock, Garden Nightshade, each 4 oz. Bittersweet 3 oz. Simmer in spirits and water to get the strength. Strain and add 18 oz lard or fresh butter. Bring to a proper consistency and apply on all tumors, which are indolent cancerous or serious and where first showing themselves to carry them away on the breast or elsewhere.

---

165 water hemlock
166 known by the common names thorn apple, jimsonweed (jimson weed) or devil's snare

62

X Spasmodic Atackts

The following forms an exelent preparation for the relief of Spasmodic Atacts viz, take of Cramp bark known as high Cranbury 2 oz Skullcap Skunk cabbage of each 1 oz cloves ½ oz Capsicum ¼ oz have all in powder coursely bruised and add 2 qts good Cherry or Nature wine doce one to two fluid ozs, three times pr day a decoction can be taken instead of the above but not so effective   B # 4 a

Syrup for the lungs X

Wahoo 2 oz. Spikenard 4 oz Elecompain 2 oz Tamerac bark not rossed or in other with the rough bark on) and dry 4 oz bloodroot 4 drachms Mandrake Root ½ oz White root 3 oz Slipery Elm bark 3 oz poplar bark 2 oz pulverize and add Alchol reduced with watter ½ for in other words reduce the Alcohol with as much watter as there is Alcohol, sufficient to cover the articles let stand 3 days puseculate the Alcohol and set by next add hot watter to the articles till the strength is extracted

Spasmodic Attacks

The following forms an excellent preparation for the relief of spasmodic attacks. Take of Cramp Bark[167] known as high cranberry 2 oz, skullcap[168], skunk cabbage of each 1 oz, cloves ½ oz, capsicum ʒij [ʒ=ounce]. Have all in powder coarsely bruised and add 2 quarts good cherry or nature wine. Dose: one to two fluid ozs, three times per day, a decoction can be taken instead of the above but not so effective. B. F. Hale

Syrup for the lungs

Wahoo 2 oz, Spikenard 4 oz, Elecampane 2 oz, Tamarack Bark not roped (or in other with the rough bark on) and dry 4 oz, bloodroot 4 drachms, mandrake root ½ oz, White root[169] 3 oz, slippery elm bark 3 oz, poplar bark 2 oz. Pulverize and add alcohol reduced with water ½ (or in other words reduce the alcohol with as much water as there is alcohol, sufficient to cover the articles). Let stand 3 days, percolate the alcohol, and set by. Next add hot water to the articles till the strength is extracted

---

167 Viburnum opulus
168 common name for *Scutellaria*, a genus of flowering plants in the mint family.
169 A common name for several plants

run over and over till clear boil to 3 pts add three pds honey one pd white sugar bring to a boiling heat throw off the scum as it rises when cool add the Spirits. Run, *that is through the percolator* shake well and to every pt add 3 drachms tinct Ipicac and the same of tinct lobelia **Dose** from one tea to a table Spoonful 3 or 4 times a day. the last on going to bed. Bathe the feet with hot watter nearely every night keep the bowels in a soluble condition. B.H. I.H.

× Dysmenorrhea or painful Menstration
Quinine 2 grs Extract Stramonium 2 grs Morphine ½ gr. Macrotin 1 gr. Hyoseyamus 2 grs mix to form 1 pill. It will be large. add quantities in proportion to form as many pills as desired one to be taken every 2 hours or as needed to procure ease when the pain comes on hard commence with the pills when the pain commences take enough to quiet the distress for. r×××i÷=

run over and over till clear. Boil to 3 pints. Add three pds honey, one pd white sugar, bring to a boiling heat. Draw off the scum as it rises. When cool add the spirits, run through the percolator, shake well and to every pint add 3 drachms tinct ipecac and the same of tinct lobelia. Dose: from one tea to a table spoonful 3 or 4 times a day, the last on going to bed. Bathe the feet with hot water nearly every night. Keep the bowels in a soluble condition. B. F. H.

Dysmenorrhea or Painful Menstruation

Quinine 2 grains, extract stramonium[170] 2 grains, morphine ½ grain, macerotin? 1 grain, Hyoscyamus[171] 2 grains. Mix to form 1 pill. It will be large. Add quantities in proportion to form as many pills as desired, one to be taken every 2 hours or as needed to produce case when the pain comes on hard, commence with the pills when the pain commences take enough to quiet the distress for fannies.[172]

---

170 Thornapple, Jimson weed or devil's snare
171 a small genus of flowering plants in the nightshade family, Solanaceae
172 Translated from code

64   Dr Hales best and
                                    Lightening
R+ Anti bilious pills, Thunder and
Podophillin, Gamboge, Shammony,
Leptandrin each (solution 70 drops)
one grain mix pill
give enough to keep a little action daily but
not to reduce the system. Alt 1 drachm
Cayenne 10 grs,

+ Cough) Syloling B # 1 Har —
Spikenard 2 oz Wid [Yarr?] 1 oz B [ ] dred 1 oz
Skunk Cabbage 1 oz Lobelia 1/2 drachm Comfrey root
1/2 oz Capsicum 1/2 drachm, Valerian or Ladyslipper
1/2 oz Elecampane 1/2 oz grind all moderately
fine add 1 pt Alcohol and 1 pt Water run off
Repeatedly and if by the first run add add
1 1/2 pts hot water let remain on roots until
cold then run off a number of times add the
first and last run together with 1 pt white
Sugar dissolve and run through 3 times and add
to every pt 2 drachms Laudanum bottle for
use (B) to the above add 2 oz Tamarac
bark or the same of white pine Bark,

Dr. Hale's best and Last Liver Pills: Thunder and Lightning

Podophyllin,[173] Gamboge, Scammony, Leptandrin[174], each one grain mix pill, Croton Oil[175] 70 drops. Give enough to keep a little action daily but not to reduce the system. Nitre 1 drachm, Cayenne 10 grains.

Cough Medicine B. F. Hale

Spikenard 2 oz, wild turnip 1 oz, bloodroot ½ oz, skunk cabbage 1 oz, lobelia ½ drachm, comfrey root ½ oz, capsicum ½ drachm, valerian or lady slipper ½ oz, elecampane ½ oz, grind all moderately fine, add 1 pint alcohol and 1 pint water. Run off repeatedly and let by the first run and add 1½ pints hot water. Let remain on roots until cold, then run off a number of times. Add the first and last—run together with 1 pint white sugar, dissolve and run through 3 times and add to every pint 2 drachms laudanum. Bottle for use A. B.
To the above add 2 oz Tamarack bark or the same of white pine bark.

---

173 a cytotoxic agent that has been used topically in the treatment of genital warts
174 A bitter glucoside obtained from plants in the genus Leptandra
175 a foul-smelling oil, formerly used as a purgative, obtained from the seeds of a tropical Asian croton tree.

× Dysenteric Diar. Cordial

Wamoo roots 4oz Little Catnip 1 oz
Peppermint plant 2 oz Geranium oz
Clanestick 2 oz Blackbury root 2 oz add spirits
to cover it. let stand 6 days prep out the Liquor
put the dregs boiling in water. let boil to get the
strength. Strain and boil very strong. Strain. Set the add
the spirit Run and add white sugar to form a
syrup with one oz Tinct Kino to every qt and the
same of Paragoric Shake well let be kept in tight
stopt Bottles to the above add 2 oz White Oak bark.
Add Oil Cynnamon 1 oz bycarbonate potash
1 oz Loaf Sugar 2 ½ oz this makes 2 qts.

× Ague Pills, by AAV

Quinine 20 grs Ipecac 65 grs Cayene 10 grs Piperine
(pure) 40 grs mix all and form 20 pills for good
size pills) and give one every 2 hours untill 5 are
taken then one every 3 hours untill 5 more are
taken, and then once 3 times each day the first
pills ____ take the Ague it seldom fails
me __ may be taken to prevent a return of the disease
_____ stopps when cooled up with the red tin to

Dysenteric Med Cordial

Strawberry leaves 4 oz, little catnip 1 oz, peppermint plant 2 oz, geranium or cranesbill[176] 2 oz, blackberry root 2 oz, add spirits to cover it, let stand 6 days. Prep out the liquor. Put the dregs boiling in water, let boil to get the strength. Strain and boil very strong. Strain, settle, add the spirit, run, and add white sugar to form a syrup with one oz tincture Kino to every quart and the same of Paregoric. Shake well, let be kept in tight stopped bottles. To the above add 2 oz White Oak bark, add Essence Cinnamon 1 oz, bicarbonate potash 1 oz, loaf sugar 26 oz. This makes 2 quarts.

Ague Pills, My Last

Quinine 20 grains, Ipecac 5 grains, Cayenne 10 grains, Prucean? (pure) 40 grains, mix all and form 20 pills (or good sized pills) and give one every 2 hours until 5 are taken, then one every 3 hours until 5 more are taken, and then one 3 times each day the first of the week the Ague 10 seldom fails. More make be taken to prevent a return of the disease. Add 10 grains extract stramonium rubbed up with the solutions to fill with.

---

176 also known as alum root, crow foot and shameface

66

✗ White Liquid Physic

½ lb Sulphate soda or sulphate of Magnesia Water 1 lb and 6 pts mix & dissolve the soda then add 2 fluid oz nitro muriatic acid & one drachm & 8 grs of Alum used to allay vomiting or nausea and a [ ] purgative also for all diseases of the liver Diarrhoea Dysentery intermittent fevers &c ℞ ℞ a tablespoonful in a gill of water every hour or two till it causes one or two evacuations ℞ Powerful nervine ✗
Ladies Slipper 1 oz valerian 1 oz stramonium ½ canabis sativa 1 oz sculcap 1 oz the fluid extract can be used or a tincture made of the roots & herbs or an infusion can be made of various gelseminum or yellow jassmine 1 oz american helabore 1 oz ℞ Gonorrhoea Infection ✗
Decoction golden seal cold infusion wilde cherry bark each 1½ oz tanic acid 30 grs Sulphate morphine dissolved in the least possible quantity Alcohol 5 grs mix inject a teaspoonful every 4 or 6 hours Another (After you have read these three look over on Page 72 one or annother and think better)
✗ Decoction golden seal one fluid oz

White Liquid Physic

½ lb sulfate soda or sulfate of magnesia, water 1 and ½ pints. Mix and dissolve the soda thin. Add 2 fluid oz of nitra muriatic acid and one drachm and 8 grains of alum. Used to allay vomiting or nausea, and a purgative also for colic diseases of the liver, diarrhea, dysentery, intermittent fevers. Dose: a table spoonful in a gill of water every hour or two till it causes one or two evacuations.

Powerful Nervine

Lady's Slipper 1 oz, valerian 1 oz, stramonium cannabis saliva 1 oz, skull cap 1 oz. The fluid extract can be used in a tincture made of the roots and herbs or an infusion can be made additions gelsemium[177] or yellow jessamine 1 oz, American hellebore 1 oz.

Gonorrhea Injection

Decoction golden seal, cold infusion, wild cherry bark each 1 and ½ oz, tannic acid 30 grains, sulfate morphine dissolved in the least possible quantity, Alcohol 5 grains. Mix. Inject a teaspoonful every 4 or 6 hours.
(After you have read these three, look over on Page 177 for another, and I think better)

Another

Decoction golden seal one fluid oz

---

177 *Gelsemium sempervirens* is a twining vine in the family Gelsemiaceae

Sulphate Zinc 3 grs use as the preceding

Dr King uses no inward medicine only salts
or cooling laxatives to reduce inflamation
depends on injections?

<u>＋ Gonorrhoea</u>

R Spirits nitre dulc ℥ij
 Bolsom copaiba   ℥j
 Oil Sweet Almonds ā ℥j spts
  turpentine aā   ℥ss
 Gum Champhor grs X
mix shake before using Dose one teaspoonful 3 times a day

<u>Bleeding of the Lungs)</u>
Oil of Fire weed 8 to 10 drops 2 a day
A decoction is likewise good,

<u>fever Sores)</u>
  White vitrol XXX grs
 Crocus martis Xl grs
1 Pt water
 for fever Sores or any
Old ulcers. this is a good Recipt
and it will not fail at any time
or place

sulfate zinc 3 grains use as the preceding.
Dr. King uses no inward medicine, only salts or cooling laxatives to reduce inflammation, depends on injections.

Gonorrhea

Rx Spirits Nitre dule[178] ℥ij [℥=ounce]
Balsam copaiba[179] ℥j
Oil sweet almonds and spirits turpentine ℥js
Gum camphor grains x
Mix, shake before using. Dose: one teaspoon for 3 times a day.

Bleeding of the Lungs

Oil of Fire Weed[180] 3 to 10 drops, 2 a day. A decoction is likewise good.

Fever Sores

White vitriol[181] xxx grains
Crocus Martis[182] xi grains
1 pint water
For fever sores or any old ulcers. This is a good recipe, and it will not fail at any time or place.

---

178 Mentioned in a number of old books, not sure what this is...
179 Copaiba balsam is a sap-like substance (oleoresin) collected from the trunk of trees that belong to the Copaifera species.
180 Chamerion angustifolium
181 Zinc sulfate
182 anhydrous ferrous sulphate (FeSo4), also known as calcined copperas.

× Stomache Cordial or
bitters, ~~for the~~ Orange peal 1 ½ oz. Gentian
root 5 drachms cinnamon 1 drachm un-
pulverised peruvian bark 2 drachms —
Gum kino 2 drachms Anice sud 2 drachms
alcohol 1 pt — Cherry bark 1 ½ oz put all
in the pt of Alcthol let stand 2 days add
watter enough to make 2 qts let stand 10
days and add 8 oz Crushed or loaf sugar
stir till desolved let settle and use as you
need. I put the drugs and alcohol after steeping
2 days in the perculator add the watter run
5 or six times through and add the sugar
desolved and run again 2 or 3 times and
bottle, press the drugs and filter and add
to the first run.

Eruption on the face
Coperas in solution apply 3 times each day
give any Alteraves 3 or 4 times a day
and attend to the liver. This is very
it has been tried by myself with perfect
sucess. You may be asured that it is good

Stomach Cordial or Bitters

Orange peel 1 and ¼ oz, gentian root 5 drachms, cinnamon 1 drachm, unpulverized Peruvian bark 2 drachms, gingko 2 drachms, anise seed 2 drachms, alcohol 1 pint, cherry bark 1½ oz. Put all in the pint of alcohol, let stand 2 days, add water, enough to make 2 quarts, let stand 10 days and add 8 oz crushed or loaf sugar, stir till dissolved. Let settle and use as you need. I put the drugs and alcohol after steeping 2 days in the percolator. Add the water, run a few times through and add the sugar, dissolve, and run again 2 or 3 times and bottle. Prep the drugs and filter and add to the first run.

Eruption on the Face

Copperas[183] in solution. Apply 3 times each day, give my alterative 3 or 4 times a day and attend to the liver. This is very, it has been tried by myself with perfect success. You may be assured that it is good.

---

183 Ferrous sulfate

X Liver Powders; by B.J. Hale

Podophilin 10 grs
Leptandrin 30 "
Sanguinarin 5 "
Goosinger 60 "
Scammony 10 "
Best African Ginger 10 grs
All well mixed & triturate half hour
and give powders according to age and
circumstances (Sic)

Liver Drops
Tinct Mandrake   ʒj
 "   Blackroot or   ʒj
Culver root
Tinct Blue flag or   ʒj
Iris versicolor   ʒj

Mix all together and give to an adult
1 teaspoonful 3 do. or 4 times every 3 & 4 hour
and increase the quantity 2 or 3 teaspoonfuls if the mouth does not become sore
or the stomach is not sickened or the bowels
not affected with pain or move too freely
Continue the medicine a good length of time

Liver Powders by B. F. Hale

Rhodphialia[184] 10 grains
Leptandrin[185] 50 grains
Sanguinarine[186] 5 grains
Loaf sugar 60 grains
Scammony 10 grains
Best African Ginger 10 grains
All well mixed, triturate half hour and give powders according to age and circumstances. It is sure.

Liver Drops

Tinct Mandrake ℥j [℥=ounce]
Tinct Blackroot ℥j
Culver Root ℥ij
Tinct Blue Flag or Iris Versicolor ℥j
Mix all together and give to an adult 1 teaspoonful 3, 4 or 5 times every 3 or 4 hours and increase the quantity 2 or 3 teaspoonfuls inf the mouth does not become sore or the stomach is not sickened, or the bowels not affected with pain or move too freely. Continue the medicine a good length of time.

---

184 Oxblood lilies
185 A bitter glucoside obtained from plants of the genus *Leptandra*
186 a toxic polycyclic ammonium ion.

And an improvement of symptoms will be nearly sirtain, (Good)

Simple Cerate ×
Lard 8 oz
White or yellow wax 4 oz
melt together and stir till cold.

Rheumatic Tinct
Wahork 2 oz, Corash 1 oz
Bloodroot Rot 1 oz
Black Cohush 2 oz
White Helibore ½ oz
Prickly Aash Burys 1 oz
Poke burys 3 oz
Rye Whiskey 1 qt
give the tinct from five to 10 minutes before eating 3 times a day.

Thet bathing drops ×
Bloodroot 1 oz
Wild turnip 1 oz
Put in (a) qt of Brandy bathe 3 times each day. N.B. Bathe upwards in every case

and improvement of the symptoms will be nearly certain. (Good).

Simple Cerate

Lard 8 oz
White or Yellow wax 4 oz
Melt together and stir till cold

Rheumatic Tinct

Wahoo 2 oz, Potash 1 oz
Bloodroot 1 oz
Black Cohosh 2 oz
White Hellebore ½ oz
Prickly Hash Berries 1 oz
Poke Berries[187] 3 oz
Rye Whiskey 1 quart
Give the tinct from five to 10 minutes before eating 3 times a day.

The Bathing drops

Bloodroot 1 oz
Wild turnip 1 oz
Put in a quart of brandy. Bathe 3 times each day A. B. Bathe upwards in any case

---

187 Pokeberry is a perennial herb

Rheumatism x

Cocash 4 oz
Black Cohush 3 oz
Prickly Aush Berries 2 oz
Blckroot 1½ oz
Alcohol 3 pts
Poke Berries 4 oz

---

x Linneament for Sprains,
Bruses Strains, Rheumatism,
Neuraliga, and for
all the cases where a
Linneament can be usefull, Toothache,
Oil of Wormwood ¼ oz
Laudanum ¼ oz
Oil Origanum ½ oz
Tinct Capsicum ¼ oz
Gum Camphor ¼ oz
Put Alcohol ennough to fill pt Bottle

Vermafuge
Oil wormseed and oil Tansy each 1 oz. Spts
Turpintine 1½ oz Castor oil 2 oz Croton oil 4 drops
Oil Annis ½ drachm Dose from ½ to 1 teaspoon

Rheumatism

Cocash? 4 oz
Black Cohosh 3 oz
Prickly Ash Berries 2 oz
Bloodroot ½ oz
Alcohol 3 pints
Poke Berries 4 oz

Liniment for Sprains, Bruises, Strains, Rheumatism, Neuralgia and for all the cases where a liniment can be useful. Toothache.

Oil of Wormwood ¼ oz
Laudanum ¼ oz
Oil Origanum ½ oz
Tinct Capsicum ¼ oz
Gum Camphor ¼ oz
Put Alcohol enough to fill pint Bottle

Vermifuge

Oil wormwood and oil Tansy[188] each 1 oz. Spirits turpentine ½ oz, Castor oil 2 oz, Croton oil 4 drops, oil anise ½ drachm. Dose: from ½ to 1 teaspoonful.

---

[188] blue tansy is harvested from tiny yellow flowers in the chamomile family

72

to be given every 3 or 4 hours till the bowels
move freely and then give smaller doses
to carry off the worms, Good,

X Gonorrhoea

Take Cannada or fir balsam one fluid
oz Spts Nitre Sweet, 4 fluid ozs oil Turpentine 2
fluid drachms powered Camphor one drachm
mix well together Dose a teaspoonful 3 times a day
when the inflamitory symptoms have been
subdued powered Kino one drachm may be
added to the above use with the above during
the inflamitory stage a tea of burdock root
and marsh mallon freely after the inflamitory
symptoms have subsided the following is very
good but very hard to take, take basam
Copaiba Sweet Spts Niter Compound
Spts lavender Tinct muriate of Iron each
one fluid oz (mix) the Dose is a teaspoonful
3 times a day shake well before taking every
time and in order to protect the teeth from
the injurious effects of the acid in the tinct
of iron wash the mouth with a solution
of Saleratus and Super Carbon of Soda,

to be given every 3 or 4 hours till the bowels move freely and then give smaller doses to carry off the worms. Good.

Gonorrhea

Take Canada or fir balsam one fluid oz. Spirits Nitre Sweet 4 fluid ozs, oil turpentine 2 fluid drachms, preserved camphor one drachm. Mix well together. Dose: a teaspoonful 3 times a day. When the inflammatory symptoms have been subdued, powdered Kino one drachm may be added to the above. Use with the above during the inflammatory stage a tea of burdock root and marshmallow freely after the inflammatory symptoms have subsided. The following is very good, but hard to take. Take balsam, copaiba, sweet spirits niter compound, spirits lavender, tinct[189] muriate of iron[190] each one fluid oz (mix). The Dose is a teaspoonful 3 times a day. Shake well before taking every time and in order to protect the teeth from the injurious effects of the acid in the tinct of iron wash the mouth with a solution of saleratus and super carbon of soda.

---

189 Tincture: A solution of alcohol or alcohol and water
190 Chloride of iron

For Tape Worm

Juice of Blue Flag with salt Salt fish Onions
Garlics & give a Purgative of mandrake every other day

Plaster for Tape Worms

Make a strong decoction of Rue Balmony Worm
wood equal parts Take equal parts of this decoction
& beefs gall add a little aloes and Asafoetida
boil the whole together to the consistence of plaster
Apply a plaster 3 inches square over the pit of the
stomach for 3 days change the plaster daily at the
end give a strong purge

X Excellent Cologne Water

Take oil lavender oil bergamont of each one fluid drachm
oil lemon oil rosemary each 2 fluid drachms oil
cloves oil cinnamon each 8 drops Alcohol one pint
if desired oil of roses & tincture of musk each
10 drops cork it tight and allow it to stand 2 weeks
before using shaking it frequently

X Carminative or Infant Cordial

Pleurisy root Sculcap Skunk cabbage hops Cramp-
bark prickly ash berries or bark Calamus angelica
Seeds Sassafras bark Catnip blows or leaves Foreign
Valerian motherwort each one ounce Cochineal 1 oz

For Tape Worm

Juice of Blue Flag with salt. Salt fish, onions, garlic and give a purgative of mandrake every other day.

Plaster for Tape Worms

Make a strong decoction[191] of Rue, Balmony[192], Wormwood equal parts. Take equal parts of this decoction and beefs gall, add a little aloe and asafetida[193]. Boil the whole together to the consistency of plaster. Apply a plaster 3 inches square over the pit of the stomach for 3 days. Change the plaster daily. At the end give a strong purge.

Excellent Cologne Water

Take oil lavender, oil bergamot, of each one fluid drachm, oil lemon, oil rosemary each 2 fluid drachms, oil cloves, oil cinnamon each 8 drops. Alcohol one pint. If desired, oil of roses and tincture of musk each 10 drops. Cork it tight and allow it to stand 2 weeks before using, shaking it frequently.

Carminative[194] or Infant Cordial

Pleurisy root[195], skull cap, skunk cabbage, hops, cramp bark, prickly ash berries or bark, calamus[196], angelica[197] suds, sassafras bark, catnip blows or leaves, foreign valerian mother wort each one ounce. Cochineal 1 oz.

---

191 the liquor resulting from concentrating the essence of a substance by heating or boiling, especially a medicinal preparation made from a plant.
192 AKA Chelone, Snake-head, Bitter Herb
193 Dried latex from Ferula, a perennial herb
194 Relieves flatulence
195 A brilliant orange flowered herb
196 Sweet Flag
197 Angelica archangelica

74

Ginger & Capsicum each ℥j pour over six pints boiling watter when cold add 3 pints good gin or other spirits use the percolater on time & decant & add 2 ℔ loaf sugar — for restless children, gripes, flatulency, wind cholic sour stomache, eases pain produses rest and quieting, removes caugh prevents morpid accumulations in the stomache.

× Worms a good Vermafuge —
Caster oil, oil wormseed each 2 oz oil turpentine one oz oil anice ½ oz oil croton 4 drops oil tansy 12 drops oil wormwood 10 drops Dose from half to one teaspoonful to have a free effect

+ Cough Med.
Bloodroot 1½ oz. Dicitalis 1 oz Chary bark 2 oz Liqurish root 2 oz Skunk cabbage 1 oz Black Cohosh 2 oz Anice sud 2 oz Valerian root 2 oz percolate the articles all mixed togather and coarsely pulverised after geting all the strength by spirits add hot water and clear the drugs perfectly and bring the watery solution down in a vapor bath to a thickness of thin syrup and add to the spirit tincture. add syrup of white sugar and to every pint add ℥j Laudinum Dose a teuspoon ful from 3 to 4 or 6

Ginger and capsicum each ʒij. Pour over six pints boiling water. When cold add 3 pints good gin or other Spirits, use the percolator on tinc and decant and add 2 lbs loaf sugar. For restless children, gripes, flatulence, wind colic, sour stomach, eases pain, produces rest and quiet naps. Removes cough, prevents mortified accumulations in the stomach.

Worms: a good Vermifuge

Castor oil, oil wormseed each 2 oz, oil turpentine one oz, oil anise ½ oz, oil croton 4 drops, oil tansy 12 drops, oil wormwood 10 drops. Dose: from half to one teaspoonful to have full effect.

Cough Med

Bloodroot 1½ oz, digitalis 1 oz, cherry bark 2 oz, licorice root 2 oz, skunk cabbage 1 oz, black cohosh, 2 oz, anise seed 2 oz, valerian root 2 oz. Percolate the articles all mixed together and coarsely pulverize after getting all the strength by spirits, add hot water and clear the dregs perfectly and bring the watery solution down in a vapor bath to a thickness of thin syrup, and add to the spirit tincture. Add syrup of white sugar and to every pint add ʒij [ʒ=ounce] laudanum. Dose a teaspoonful from 3 to 4 or 6 times a day a very little time Lobelia 1℥ to the pint

Lip Salve

Oil almonds 3 oz oil olive 1 oz spermaceti 2 oz white wax 1 oz melt all together & color with anchura root powdered & tied in a bag & kept in the mixture while melting after cooling a little add 10 or 12 drops otto rose or burgamont

For Cough

Caster or good sweet oil 1 oz 4 table spoon fulls of loaf sugar or honey and the juice of two good lemons gently simmer all together Dose discretionary

Eye Wash

6 oz of rectifyed spts wine dissolved ℥j Gum Camphor then add two small handfulls dried Elder flowers let steep 24 or 48 hours this is superior to any now in use

To remove Films

Equal parts saltpetre loaf sugar & rock salt ¼ part as much alum pulverised as fine as possible mixed with honey reduce with rain water

Sticking salve

12 oz rasin Bees wax mutton tallow each 1 oz melt and pour in to cold water

times a day, a very little lobelia 1ʒ [ounce] to the pint.

Lip Salve

Oil almonds 3 oz, oil olive 1 oz, spermaceti 2 oz, white wax 1 oz. Melt all together and color with an ?? root powdered and tied in a bag and kept in the mixture while melting after cooling a little. Add 10 or 12 drops of the rose or bergamot.

For Cough

Castor or good, sweet oil 1 oz, 4 tablespoonfuls of loaf sugar or honey and the juice of five good lemons gently simmer altogether. Dose discretionary.

Eye Wash

6 oz of rectified spirits wine dissolved ʒj [ʒ=ounce], gum camphor, then add two small handfuls dried elder flowers, let steep 24 or 48 hours. This is superior to any now in use.

To remove Films

Equal parts saltpeter, loaf sugar and rock salt, ¼ part as much alum pulverized as fine as possible, mixed with honey. Reduce with rain water.

Sticking Salve

12 oz rosin, bees wax, mutton tallows each 1 oz and pour into cold water.

76

~~Hum Syrup~~

✕ Dr Hales Cholera Syrup.
Tinct Rheubarb   1 pt
Tinct Opium   6 oz
"   Lobelia   6 oz
"   Murrh   8 oz
"   Cayenne   4 oz
Oil   Peppermint   1 oz
Carbonate potapa   1 oz
Symple ~~that~~ Syrup   1 qt
Mix, good medicine.

✕ Black Linneament
Olive oil   1½ oz
Sylphuric Acid   1 drachm
Mix well together and add ½ oz Spts
Turpentine. an active counter irritant
but does not Vesicle ^means^ rais the skin,
to be rubed on 2 a day untill the Skin
becomes tender and inflamed. used in
indolent swellings. Swelling of joints
Rheumatic pains &c

Dr. Hale's Cholera Syrup

Tinct Rhubarb 1 pint
Tinct Opium 6 oz
Tinct Lobelia 6 oz
Tinct Myrrh 8 oz
Tinct Cayenne 4 oz
Oil Peppermint 1 oz
Carbonate Potash 1 oz
Simple Syrup 1 quart
Mix. Good Medicine

Black Liniment

Olive oil 1½ oz
Sulfuric Acid 1 drachm
Mix well together and ad ½ oz spirits turpentine.
An active counter irritant but does not vesicle (means raise the skin), to be rubbed on 2 a day until the skin becomes tender and inflamed. Used in indolent swellings, swelling of joints, rheumatic pains.

℞ Pomade for restoring the hair, B. E. ##

Pulverised Cantharides   ʒj
Rectified spts wine   ʒviij

Macerate 12 days filter mix 10 parts of this tinct with 90 parts of cold lard adding oil Burgamont or any other kind perfumary in 99 cases out of 100 if the medicine is continued the hair will be restored,

X Nervine and Carminitive Balsam
Peony 2 oz. Catnip 1 oz. Skulcap 3 oz. ladys lipes 3 oz. Skunk cabbage 2 oz. Angelica Root ½ oz. Calamus Root ½ oz. Caraway Cardamen and Annis seed each ½ oz. Perculate. Run off 1 qt By repeated runnings with diluted Alcohol set by and add hot water and run till the strength is extracted and boil the water runnings down to 1 pt add it while the sperit runnings is made hot and the water running is liquise hot together and deselve one ptt loaf suger in it when cold add 2 oz Paragoric Gum Campher ʒij B. E. ##

Pomade for restoring the hair, B. F. H.

Pulverized cantharides ℥j [℥=ounce]
Rectified spirits wine ℥j
Macerate 12 days, filter rum 10 parts of this tinct with 90 parts of cold lard, adding oil bergamot or any other kind perfume. In 99 cases out of 100 if the medicine is continued the hair will be restored.

Nervine and Carminative Balsam

Peony 2 oz, catnip 1 oz, skull cap 3 oz, lady's slipper 3 oz, skunk cabbage 2 oz, Angelica root ½ oz, calamus root ½ oz, caraway, cardamom[198], and anise seed each ½ oz.
Percolate, run off 1 quart. By repeated runnings with diluted alcohol set by and add hot water and run till the strength is extracted and boil the water runnings down to 1 pint—add it while the spirit runnings is made hot and water running is liquid hot together and dissolve one pint loaf sugar. In it when cold add 2 oz Paregoric gum camphor ℈ij [℈=scruple]. B.F.H.

---

198 a spice made from the seeds of several plants in the genera Elettaria and Amomum in the family Zingiberaceae.

78

Conklin's Salve

Rozin 12 oz, Beeswax Mutton tallow each 1 oz melt together work it in rolls in cold water.

Lord's Salve

Mutton tallow 1 pd Beeswax and white turpentine each ¼ pd meld together and add finely powered virdigris one tablespoonful. Good / these drops are good after just such as be left at Home

Cholera drops

1 pt and ½ best brandy 2 oz Spts camphor ½ oz prickly ash berries 1 oz laudanum 1 oz molasses ½ oz cayenne 1 oz myark mix let stand 1 week filter. Dose from a tea to a tablespoonful Good.

For injection in Leucorrhoea Gonorrhoea and to wash the   in Gonorrhoea. Laudanum   Gutta 40
    Gum arabic grs 12
    S Lead   grs 8
    Sulph zinc   grs 4
    Rose water   8 z

Conklin's Salve

Rosin 12 oz, Beeswax, Mutton Tallow each 1 oz. Melt together, work it in rolls on cold water.

Lord's Salve

Mutton tallow 1 pd, Beeswax and white turpentine each ½ pd, meld together and add finely powdered verdigris one tablespoonful. Good.

Cholera Drops

(these drops are grandfather's best—such as he left at home)
1 pint and ½ best brandy, 2 oz spirits camphor, 2 oz prickly ash berries, 1 oz laudanum, 1 oz molasses, ½ oz cayenne,
1 oz myrrh. Mix. Let stand 1 week. Filter. Dose: from a tea to a tablespoonful. Good.
For injection in Leukorrhea, Gonorrhea and to wash the head or the penis[199] in Gonorrhea.
Laudanum Gutta 3o
Gum Arabic grains 12
S. Lead grains 8
Sulfur Lime grains 4
Rose Water 8 oz

---

199 Translated from code

X Pain killer ℞ # 14 o..

Alcohol 1 gall Gum Camphor ℥v
Oil Organum Hemlock each ℥v
Oil Terpentine Tinct Coyonne ℥ij
Oil Sasafras Peppermint Spearmint each ℥ij
Laudanum ℥ij mix use externaly and
Internaly. Doce from 10 to 60 drops for
Acute Rheumatism and Chronic. nervious
spasims stiffness of joints chilblanes swellings
of all kinds add to the above Musk,
For Goitre swelled X / Take of Iodine
neck Scrofulous tumors (Hydriodate Potash
tumors, (or Potash ℥ij
desolve in 2½ oz water apply it with a feather
continue its use twice a day untill the
tumor disapears if the parts become to tender
by its use it can be omytted a single day
onely then use again it should cause the
scarfskin to peal off which it will do a number
of times before the tumor will entirely
disapear it is not neasary to soak it in mearly
witting the skin night and morning will be
sufficent the above will be very useful to

Pain Killer—B. F. Hale

Alcohol 1 gallon, gum camphor ℥v [℥=ounce]
Oil Origanum, hemlock each ℥v
Oil Turpentine, Tinct Cayenne ℥j
Oil Sassafras, Peppermint, Spearmint each ℥jj
Laudanum ℥jj
Mix. Use externally and internally. Dose: from 10 to 60 drops for Acute Rheumatism and chronic nervous spasms, stiffness of joints, chilblains, swellings of all kinds. Add to the above myrrh.

For Goiter Swelled Neck, Scrofulous Cancers, Tumors

Take of Iodine ℥j [℥=ounce], Hydriodate potash[200] or potash ℥j, dissolve in 2½ oz water, apply it with a feather. Continue its use twice a day until the tumor disappears. If the parts become too tender by its use, it can be omitted a single day. Only then use it again. It should cause the scar skin to peel off, which it will do a number of times before the tumor will entirely disappear. It is not merely to rub it in, merely wetting the skin night and morning will be sufficient—the above will be very useful to

---

200 Possibly the chemical compound KOI

apply over any part of the body where there
is either pain or swelling. B H Hall

P.S. while applying the Iodine &c externaly
arse a powerful alterative with ½ oz
Iodine of Potasium with one pt of the
altative. Doce a tea spunful ⅔ to
each meal.

Colyrium or ⎫ 1 table spoonful each of tosh
Eye Watter × ⎬ Salt and white Vitriol heat
on copper or earthen or glass until it is dry
add blue vitriol the size of a pea one
2 punful of white sugar (loaf) pulverize
put in ½ pt soft watter if to strong reduce
with more watter. Laudanum 2 oz
Diarrhoea & × ⎫ Spts Camphor   ,,
Colera morbus × ⎬ E&̃ Pepermint   ,,
Hoofmans anodine 2 oz Tinct Cayenne 2
drachms Tinct Ginger 1 oz mix Doce
one tea spunful in a strong tea of peppermint or brandy a table spoonful to be
repeated every hour — but the doce for children must be less in propotion to age —
it is good to appy externaly to restor action if cold
takes place in Diarrhoea or Cholera morbus. B H H

apply over any part of the body where there is either pain or swelling. B. F. Hale

P. S. While applying the Iodine externally use a powerful alterative with ½ oz Iodine of potassium with one pint of the alterative. Dose: a teaspoonful after each meal.

Collyrium[201] or Eye Matter

1 tablespoonful each of table salt and white vitriol. Heat on copper or earthen or glass until it is dry. Add blue vitriol the size of a pea, one spoonful of white sugar (loaf) pulverize, put in ½ pint soft water. If too strong reduce it with more water.

Diarrhea and Cholera Morbus

Laudanum 2 oz
Spirits camphor 2 oz
Essence Peppermint 2 oz
Hoffman's anodyne[202] 2 oz
Tinct Cayenne 2 drachms
Tinct Ginger 1 oz. Mix.

Dose: one teaspoonful in a strong tea of peppermint or brandy, a tablespoonful to be repeated every hour—but the dose for children must be less in proportion to age. It is good to apply externally to restore action if coldness takes place in diarrhea or Cholera Morbus. B.F.H.

---

201 Tetrahydrozoline
202 Hoffman's Anodyne was a compound sometimes known as "Spirit of Ether", produced through a process of distillation. It is a solution of one part diethyl ether in three parts alcohol.

Salt-Rhume Ointment

boil tobacco strong add 1 table spoonful
tar 1 ditto spts turpentine
1 " Sulphur 1 of ginger 1 of alspice
1 black pepper Lard 'n get boil well together

Pills for Dropsy

Jalap 30 grs Gamboge 30 grs soap 20
grs Podophillin 2 grs Cayenne 35 grs
Croton oil 90 drops mix with thick solution
gum tragacanth at the same time use
freely of a tea made of queen of the meadow
or sweet elder bark, dwarf elder roots
with cream tartar and carbonate of potash
disolved in it ℞ Spanish flies ʒiij
Emmenagogue Blue cohush root 2 oz
Tinct — X Ergot and Smart Weed
each 1 oz Mandrake root ½ oz Black
Helabor ½ oz Strong Solution Borax 1 oz
oil Savine 1 fluid oz Alcohol one pt and
3 gills tinct the first five articles 12 days
filter and add the solution Borax and
oil Savin Doce a tea spoonful if the stomach
and bowels will bear it 3 times a day ℞

Salt-Rhume Ointment

Boil tobacco strong. Add 1 tablespoonful tar, 1 ditto? Spirits Turpentine, 1" sulfur, 1 of ginger, 1 of allspice, 1 black pepper, lard ½ pd, boil well together.

Pills for Dropsy

Jalap 30 grains, Gamboge 30 grains, soap 20 grains, Podophyllin 20 grains, Cayenne 33 grains, Croton oil 90 drops. Mix with thick solution gum tragacanth[203], at the same time use freely a tea made of queen of the meadow[204], sweet elder bark, dwarf elder roots, with cream tartar and carbonate of potash dissolved in it. B. F. H.

Emmenagogue

Spanish flies ʒijj [ʒ=ounce], blue cohosh root 2 oz, ergot and smart weed each 1 oz, mandrake root ½ oz, black hellebore ¼ oz, strong solution borax 1 oz, oil savin[205] ½ fluid oz, alcohol one pint and 3 gills tinct the first five articles. 12 days filter and the solution Borax and oil savin. Dose: A teaspoonful if the stomach and bowels will bear it 3 times a day. B. F. Hale

---

[203] a natural gum obtained from the dried sap of several species of Middle Eastern legumes of the genus *Astragalus*,
[204] *Filipendula ulmaria*, commonly known as meadowsweet or mead wort
[205] Savin oil is extracted from Juniperus sabina

82

Spice Bitters

Gentien Root 1 lb. Orrange peel 1 lb
Red Sanders 4 oz Cinnamon and
and ginger each 4 oz Black pepper 1 oz
mix all well and to every 2 oz add one
quart watter boil to one pt strain
add ½ pt Loaf Sugar and 1 pt rum or
Brandy as the case may be for a tonic
to restore appetite streghen digestion give
general tonic to the system to be taken
after after moveing the bowels with my
mild croton pills.

Cutaneous) Burnt Allum ʒij citric
Cancers } or tartaric acid ʒij Oxalic
to be tride for } acid ʒij rain watter ½
tetter Ringworm) pt. to be applyed with a
warts moles cornes &c }
     Cammal hair pencil. B, H, H

Comp tinct) Oil organum Hemlock
Camphor } aa (this means) equal parts ½ pt) Oil
   × Sassafras Oil Cajeput aa ʒij
tinct Cayenne 2 oz mix for a linneament
to stimulate for all kinds of pains.

Spice Bitters

Gentian root 1 lb, orange peel 1 lb, Red Saunders 4 oz, cinnamon and ginger each 4 oz, black pepper 1 oz. Mix all well and to every 2 oz add one quart water. Boil to one pint—strain, add ½ pint loaf sugar and 1 pint rum or brandy as the case may be for a tonic to restore appetite, strengthen digestion, give general tonic to the system to be taken after moving the bowels with my mild croton pills.

Cutaneous Cancers

to be tried for tetter[206], Ringworm, warts, moles, corns. Burnt alum ℥j [℥=ounce], citric or tartaric acid ℥ij, Oxalic acid[207] ℥ij, rain water ½ pint. To be applied with a camel hair pencil. B.F.H.

Comp Tinct Camphor

Oil Origanum, hemlock (aa) this means equal parts, ½ lb Oil Sassafras, Oil Cajeput aa, tinct Cayenne. Mix for a liniment to stimulate for all kinds of pains,

---

206 any skin condition characterized by reddish vesicular eruptions and intense itching
207 Oxalic acid is an organic compound with the formula $C_2H_2O_4$

Pery Davises Pain Killer

Camphor ʒiiʒ Gum Mynh ʒß. Goac
gum ʒij Caynne ʒß Alcohol 1 pt Spts
turpentine ʒij Laudanum 1½ oʒ

Kitridge nerve) Cicuta Leaves 4 oz tobacco
Ointment x) 2oz Yellow dock 4oz yarget
root 4oz Stramonium Leaves 4oz Deadly
night shade 4oz Bittersweet bark 8oz extract the strength and boil down to the
consistance of an ointment 1 lb and 2 oz
hogs lard simmer well together. used
for stiff joints sprains bruises and for
cancerous lumps, Scrofulous swellings
a great discutient,

Bone Linneament) 4oz Organum oil
1 gill neatsfoot oil ½ pt beefs gall ½ pt
alcohol Camphor 4 oz gum) disolve
the camphor in the alcohol add the oil
Organum the neats foot oil and the gall
Shake well together,

Pery Davises Pain Killer

Camphor ℥js [℥=ounce], Gum Myrrh ℥js Guaiac Gum ℥ij, Cayenne ℥js, Alcohol 1 pint, Spirits turpentine ℥ij Laudanum ½ oz

Kitridge Nerve Ointment

Cicuta leaves 2 oz, tobacco 2 oz, yellow dock 4 oz, garget root 4 oz, stramonium leaves 4 oz, deadly nightshade 4 oz, bittersweet bark 3 oz. Extract the strength and boil down to the consistency of all ointment 1 pd and 2 oz hog's lard. Simmer well together. Used for stiff joints, sprains, bruises, and for cancerous lumps, scrofulous swellings, a great discutient.[208]

Bone Liniment

1 oz Origanum oil, 1 gill neatsfoot oil, ½ pint beefs gall, 1 pint alcohol (camphor ½ oz gum). Dissolve the camphor in the alcohol, add the oil Origanum, the neatsfoot oil and the gall. Shake well together.

---

208 An agent (as a medicinal application) which serves to disperse morbid matter.

84.

Scrofula Pill

Take of Iodine grs 50 Sulphate of Morphia 10 grs burnt Spunge grs 100 triturate these well together into fine powder from the pill mass divide into 100 pills to be kept in a dry place Dose 2 or 3 pills every day

Com tinct Camphor ⎫ Gum Myrrh 4 oz
Rheumatic drops ⎬ Alcohol 1 gall
Or Pain Killer   ⎭ Pulverize fine African Cayenne 2 oz tinct the above 14 days filter and to every gall add Camphor 4 oz oil of Organum and oil Hemlock each 1 lb Oil Sasafras and Oil Cage put each 2 oz Spts turpentine 1 oz use in every painful affliction Chronic Rheumatism Bruises Sprains Chilblains contusions lameness toothache Colds and Coughs Asthma and phthizic Piles Kidney Complaints pain in the head fever and Ague burnes and canker weak stomach painters colic broken

Scrofula Pill

Take of Iodine grains 30, sulfate of morphea 10 grains, burnt sponge grains 100, triturate[209] these well together into fine powder. From the pill mass divide it into 100 pills to be kept in a dry place. Dose: 2 or 3 pills every day.

Corn Tinct Camphor Rheumatic Drops

Gum Myrrh 4 oz, alcohol 1 gall, pulverize fine African cayenne 2 oz, tinct the above 14 days. Filter and to every gall add camphor 4 oz, oil of Origanum and oil Hemlock each 1 lb, oil Sassafras and oil Cajeput—each 2 oz, spirits turpentine 1 oz. Use in every painful affliction, chronic rheumatism, bruises, sprains, chilblains, contusions, sameness toothache, colds and coughs, asthma and phthisic piles[210], kidney complaints, pain in the head, fever, and ague burns and canker; weak stomach, painter's colic, broken

---

209 Grind to a fine powder
210 A progressively wasting disease

breast - bowels complaint - Cholera
Cholera Morbous liver complaint
Dyspepsia, White Swellings. Good

By B. W. Hall M D

Chilblains ℞ Pure tinct Capsicum 4 parts
And strogest essence pepper-
mint 1 part mix to be rubed on the part
untill a strong tingling and electriol
feeling is produced continue daily till
well relief will be experienced the first
application 3 or 4 times effects a cure

Dr Allens } Tinct Rhei one pt Tinct
Cholera   } Myerh ʒvi Tinct Capsicum
Syrup   } ʒij Tinct Opi ʒvi Tinct
Campher ʒvi Tinct Lobelia
ʒv oil Peppermint ʒfs Carbonate Potash
ʒfs Simple Syrup 4 pts mix Dose
a tea spoonful. Good

breast, bowels complaint, cholera, cholera morbus, liver complaint, dyspepsia, white swellings. Good. By B. F. Hale

Chilblains

Pure tinct capsicum 4 parts and strongest essence peppermint 1 part. Mix. To be rubbed on the part until a strong tingling and electrical feeling is produced. Continue daily till well. Relief will be experienced. The first application 3 or 4 times effects a cure.

Dr. Allen's Cholera Syrup

Tinct Rue? one pint, tinct myrrh ℥vi [℥=ounce], tinct capsicum ℥ij, tinct opi(um?) ℥vi, tinct camphor ℥ivi, tinct lobelia ℥v, oil peppermint ℥js, carbonate potash ℥js, simple syrup 2 pints. Mix. Dose: a teaspoonful. Good.

86

Comp Ointment Stramonium

Take Bark of the root of Bittersweet Stramonium leaves Cicuta leaves Deadly nightshade Yellow dock root each 2 oz Lard 1 pd venis turpentine 2 oz bruise the whole except the turpentine if the herbs are dry cover with watter and simmer the watter out but use no spirits.) let the watter stand on the herbs 4 hours then simmer out by gentle heat add the lard simmered to a crisp strain press through linnen add the Venis turpentine Stir till cold the above medicine can be made of the ointment of the above ointments if in haist to use it — Uses. Discutient for scroffula indolent tumors all glandular swellings & tumors it should be rubed in each time 20 minutes and covered with a bandage. End

+ Tobacco 2 oz

+ Compound Wine of Comfry

take comfry Root Solomon seal Spikenard each 1 oz Canomile Calumbo gentian each ½ oz Shery 4 pts place the herbs in

Comp Ointment Stramonium

Take bark of the root of bittersweet, stramonium leaves, cicuta leaves, deadly nightshade, yellow dock root each 2 oz, lard 1 pd, Venice turpentine 2 oz. Bruise the whole except the turpentine. If the hearts are dry, cover with water and simmer the matter out but use no spirits. Let the matter stand on the herbs 4 hours, then simmer out by gentle heat. Add the lard simmered to a crisp, strain the press through linen, add the Venice turpentine, stir till cold. In the above medicine can be made of the ointment above ointments if in haste to use it. Uses: Discutent for scrofula, indolent tumors, all glandular swellings, and tumors. It should be rubbed in each time 20 minutes and covered with a bandage. End.

Compound Wine of Comfrey

Take comfrey root, Solomon Seal, spikenard, each 1 oz, chamomile, columbo, gentian each ½ oz, sherry 4 pints, place the herbs over the fire in a propper vessel cover with water let them macerate 24 hours closely covered then add the wine let stand often shakeing for 7 days & fitter Malaga wine will answer Use a valuable tonic in all female weakness Leucorrhoea Amenorrhoea weakness of the back. Good For Cough

Flowers benzian ℥j Syrup of tolu. ʒij tinct lobelia ʒj tinct Blood Root ʒij Morphine grs 1 mucelage gum arabic ʒj. Dose a tea spoonful every 2 or 3 hours. Good — End.

Nerve and Bone Linneament } Oil Organum 1 lb
Oil Rosemary 1 lb
Olive oil 2 lb. tinct Cantharides ½ lb
Spts turpentine ½ lb Strongest spts Camphor 1 oz mix all well for scrofula Inflamation chronic Rheumatism wound on man or beast Scalds Sprains bruises Contractions of chords and sinews and even to bathe the palpebra angles of the eyes in case of inflamed or sore eyes. Good (End of page)

the fire in a proper vessel cover with water. Let them macerate 24 hours, closely covered, then add the wine. Let stand, often shaking for 7 days and filter. Malaga wine will answer. Use: a valuable tonic in all female weakness, leukorrhea, amenorrhea, weakness of the back. Good.

For Cough

Flowers benzian[211] ℈ji [℈=scruple], Syrup of tolu ℥ij [℥=ounce], tinct lobelia ℥j, tinct bloodroot, ℥ij, morphine grains 1, mucilage, gum Arabic ℥j. Dose: a teaspoonful every 2 or 3 hours. Good. End.

Nerve and Bone Liniment

Oil origanum 1 lb, oil rosemary 1 lb, olive oil 2 lbs, tinct cantharides ½ lb, sprits turpentine ½ lb, strongest spirits camphor 1 oz. Mix all well for scrofula, inflammation, chronic rheumatism, wound on man or beast, scalds, sprains, bruises, contractions of chords and sinews, and even to bathe the palpebra muscles of the eyes[212] in case of inflamed or sore eyes. Good. (End of page)

---

211 unidentified
212 The levator palpebrae superioris is the muscle in the orbit that elevates the superior (upper) eyelid.

88

Dyspeptic Powders X Rs

take Poplar bark 2 lbs Golden Seal 4 oz
Cayenne 1 oz Brown Sugar 4 lbs add 1 oz
essence Pennyroyal mix thoroughly good
for Dyspepsia Costiveness afflictions of the
liver and general debility. Superior remedy
good distresses loss of appetite faintness of
the stomach Souverign remedy for Dyspepsia if Persevered in Doce a tea spoonful
in wine or warm watter three to five times
a day

Cutaneous Ointment Olive or Almond oil ℥ij

Spermaciti ʒ iii perfume to your
likeing — Add to yes Cur Rub internaly
for sores on the breast. B H¹ Hol
x Cough balsam fir balsam 2 oz honey 1 oz alcohol
1 Pt let stand closely covered 10 days Shaking it often
then filter and add 3 gills tinct Lobelia Doce from
½ to a tea spoonful several times a day good
for coughs asthma pain in the breast cramp
gravel Dropsy ghanorrhoea fluor albus
and nervous afflictions   B H¹ Hol

Dyspeptic Powders

Take poplar bark 2 lbs, golden seal 4 oz, cayenne 1 oz, brown sugar 4 lbs, add ½ oz essence pennyroyal[213], mix thoroughly. Good for dyspepsia, costiveness[214], afflictions of the liver and general debility. Superior remedy food distresses, loss of appetite, faintness of the stomach. Sovereign remedy for dyspepsia[215] if preserved in. Dose: a teaspoonful in wine or warm water three to five times a day.

Cutaneous Ointment

Olive or Almond oil ℥ji [℥=ounce], Spermaceti ℥iii, perfume to your likening = add 10 grains cur(?). Rub internally for sores on the breast. B. F. Hale

Cough Balsam

Fir balsam 1 oz, honey 1 oz, alcohol 1 pint, let stand closely covered 10 days shaking it often, then filter and add 3 gills tinct lobelia. Dose: from ½ to a teaspoonful several times a day. Good for coughs, asthma, pain in the breast, cramps, gravel, dropsy, gonorrhea, fluor albus[216], and nervous afflictions. B. F. Hale.

---

213 A mint
214 Costiveness – an unnatural retention of the fecal matter of the bowels; constipation.
215 indigestion
216 leukorrhea

Lavender Water ℞

Oil Lavender Oil bergament āā ʒiii
Otto Rose cloves āā gutta vi, musk grsii
Oil Rosemary ʒi Honey ʒj. Benzoic acid
ℨii Rectified Spts ʒvj ℔ distilled water
ʒiii mix and after standing a sufficient
length of time (the longer the better) filter
this perfume may be employed for
centing (Spts washes) *this means* or put in Linn-
ament or anything where there is a bad
smell espeially for the ladies) but is Prin-
cipaly for the toilet N b put this in no
medicine for internal uses B.H.W.
Hungary Spt Lavender ℥xii
Water] . . Rosemary ℥iv mix

good for faintness and for stimulating linneament. B.H.E.H.ab

Palpitation) Take Conium
Maculatum Ipicac āā mix form
into common sized pills Dose from 1 to 2
every 2 hours untill nausea is produced
~~those living in the country and not~~

Lavender Water

Oil lavender, oil bergamot aa ʒiii [ʒ=ounce], Otto Rose, cloves aa, gutta vi, musk grains ii, oil Rosemary ʒl Honey ʒj. Benzoic acid Ɜii, rectified spirits one pint distilled water ʒiii. Mix and after standing a sufficient length of time (the longer the better) filter this perfume. May be employed for scenting (this means spirits washes) (or put in liniment or anything where there is a bad smell especially for the ladies) but is principally for the toilet. No put this in the medicine for internal uses. B. F. H.

Hungary Water

Spirits lavender ʒxii [ʒ=ounce], rosemary ʒiv, mix. Good for faintness and for stimulating liniment. B. F. Hale

Palpitation

Take conium maculatum[217], Ipecac aa, Mix, form into common sized pills. Dose: from 1 to 2 every 2 hours until nausea is produced.

---

[217] Poison Hemlock

℞ Bitters ℔ꝶ. 74

Quassia ℥i Orange peel ℥ii Red Saunders ℥ii Cloves ℥i Cinnamon ℥i Corriander seed ℥i — Spts 2 qts steep 7 days agitate often strain through flannel —

Ointment for the eye } White vitrol 2 tea spoonfuls new honey 2 tea spoonfuls Lard 1 tea spoonfuls melt the lard and vitrol together and add the honey and Stir till cold

Cough Drops } tinct Blood root ℥i
Skunk cabbage ℥i wine of Ipicac ℥i wine of antinony ℥ß
Syrup of wild chery ℥iiij tinct Spikenard ℥ß
Parigoric ℥j — mix Syrup Squills ℥i Tinct lobelia ℥ß
Tinct Digitalis ℥i

Rx Bitters—B. F. H.

Quassia[218] ℥i[℥=ounce], orange peel ℥ii, Red Saunders, ℥ii, cloves ℥i, cinnamon ℥i, coriander seed ℥i, Spirits 2 quarts, steep 7 days, agitate often, strain through flannel.

Ointment for the eye

White vitriol 2 teaspoonfuls, new honey 2 teaspoonfuls, lard 1 teaspoonful, melt the lard and vitriol together and the honey and stir till cold.

Cough Drops

Tinct bloodroot ℥i [℥=ounce], skunk cabbage ℥i, wine of spicae ℥i, wine of antimony ℥j, syrup of wild cherry ℥iijj, tinct of spikenard ℥j, paregoric ℥j. Mix syrup squab? ℥i, tinct lobelia ½ oz, tinct digitalis ℥i.

---

218 Bitterwood

Cough Drops R⁄

Tinct Blood Root —
" Skunk cabbage = Tinct Lobelia
Wine of Ipicac
Wine " Antimony = Tinct snake Root
Tinct Spikenard
~~Hive Syrup~~ do not put this in B. F. H.
Tinct — Digitalis
Parigoric mix all and add to every oz
of th above two ʒ of syrup of wild cherry
or Beeches pulmonary balsam or my
Hellenium Balsam Doce from a tea
to a table spoonful, in active stages of a
cough the balsam Hellenium is better than
the syrup of cherry. Take 1 oz of each of
these articles.

Cough powders } Wild turnip ʒij Skunk
cabbage ʒij Blood Root
ʒij Cayenne Ɖj Lobelia Ɖij foreign or
native Ipicac Ɖij — Fox glove ʒj Lady
slipper ʒj Opium ʒj comfry ʒj Pulverize
all fine pass through gauze mix Doce
from 10 to 30 grs. Pro Rator Elecampane 6 ʒ

Liquorice ʒij

Cough Drops Rx

Tinct Bloodroot, skunk cabbage, tinct lobelia, wine of ipecac, wine of antimony, tinct snake root, tinct spikenard, ~~Hive syrup do not put~~ this in B.F.H., tinct digitalis, paregoric. Mix all and add to every oz of the above two oz of syrup of wild cherry, or Beech's pulmonary balsam or my Helenium balsam. Dose: from a teaspoonful to a tablespoonful. In active stages of a cough the balsam Helenium is better than the syrup of cherry. Take 1 oz of each of these articles.

Cough Powders

Wild Turnip ℥iij [℥=ounce], skunk cabbage ℥iij, bloodroot ℥iij, cayenne ℈j, lobelia ℈ij, foreign or native ipecac ℈ij, foxglove ℥j, lady slipper ℥j, opium ℥j, comfrey ℥j, Pulverize all fine, pass through gauze, mix. Dose: from 10 to 30 grains. Pro Rator elecampane 6 oz.

92

For Cholera. Cholera Morbous to aid in Darrhoea Dysintary. to be used with or after Beach Dysinteric Cordial, Oil cazepud Peppermint Anise cloves and as much Alcohol as of all the other articles when mixed together Doce from 16 to 50 drops according to the urgency of the case to be given in Brandy sling   Plaster ℞ ℔ ℥ ʒ

Rosin 6 oz Mutton tallow 2 oz Bole Armanium 1 oz Campfor ½ oz Cayenne ½ oz melt the tallow and Beswax add the cayne and simmer a few minutes then add the campor made fine stir well and pour into cold watter and pull it as you should wax   Good

Linneament for people
Oil Organum   2 oz
Spts Turpentine   1 oz
Olive oil   1 oz
Oil Hemlock   1 oz
Alcohol sufficient to cut the oils
or

Organum   ʒii
Spts Turpentine ʒii
hemlock   ʒi
This is a very good for hurts on men or beast good for all strains bruises and swellings on man or beast. the right hand is for the beast—

Beswax 2 oz

For Cholera, Cholera Morbus

To aid in diarrhea, dysentery. To be used with or after Beich Dysenteric cordial. Oil cajeput, peppermint, anise, cloves and as much alcohol as of all the other articles when mixed together. Dose from 16 to 50 drops according to the urgency of the case. To be given in Brandy sling.

Plaster Rx B.F.H.

Rosin 16 oz, mutton tallow 2 oz, Bole Armanium[219] 1 oz, camphor ½ oz, cayenne, ½ oz. Melt the tallow and beeswax, add the cayenne, and simmer a few minutes, then add the camphor made fine, stir well, and pour into cold water and pull it as you should wax. Good.

Liniment for People

Oil origanum 2 oz, spirits turpentine 1 oz, olive oil 1 oz, oil hemlock 1 oz. This is a very good for hurts on men or beast. Alcohol sufficient to cut the oils good for all strains, bruises, and swellings on man or beast.

---

[219] an earthy clay, usually red, native to Armenia

Sure cure for Hydrophobia

Take emediatly warm vinegar or tipid water wash the wound clean therewith then dry it then pour into the wound a few drops of Hydro Chloric acid this is sure —

Corns} 2 oz gum Amoniac 2 oz yellow wax 6 drachms Viridigris melt together spread on soft leather pare the corn keep the plaster on two weeks

For piles} Take Stramonium Ointment or fresh butter or lard mix very finely pulverized blood root enough with it to change the collor a little and add a little oil fireweed mix all well and apply morning and evening to the deseased part at the same time move the bowels gently with cream tarter and Sulpher 2 parts cream tarter and one of Sulpher

Sure Cure for Hydrophobia

Take immediately warm vinegar or tepid water, wash the wound clean therewith, then dry it. Then pour into the wound a few drops of hydrochloric acid. This is sure.

Corns

2 oz gum ammoniac, 2 oz yellow wax, 6 drachms verdigris, melt together, spread on soft leather. Pare the corn. Keep the plaster on two weeks.

For Piles

Take Stramonium ointment or fresh butter or lard, mix very finely pulverized bloodroot enough with it to change the color a little and add a little oil fireweed, mix all well and apply morning and evening to the diseased part, at the same time move the bowels gently with cream tartar and sulfur, 2 parts cream tartar and one of sulfur. B. F. H.

94

For one qt of Hellenium
Balsam, B H Hale

BloodRoot ʒiiii comfry ʒiiii
Digitalis ʒi Liquorice root ʒiiii
Squills ʒii chery Bark ℥6.
Elecampane ʒiiii, hoarhoun ʒiii
Spikenard ℥6. White Root ℥6. boil and
pour off to git full strength strain add
one pd Muskovado Sugar bring to
a boil through off the scum let cool
add Sperits Vitea 2 ounces Rum or
gin ½ pt in hot weather and one
gill in cold weather yet a gill of
the best of Rum or gin will keep
it in all kinds of weather

For Neuralgia} Tinct Nux vomica ʒij
× ×   Strichnine grs ii
Sulphate Morphea grs ii Doce from
5 to 10 drops every six hours give 10
grs carbonate of Iron 3 times a
day before eating, this is very good
try it and I do not think it will
fail   B H Hale

For one Quart of Helenium Balsam B. F. Hale

Bloodroot ℥iiii [℥=ounce], comfrey ℥iii, digitalis ℥ii, licorice root ℥iiiii, squills[220] ℥iii, cherry bark ℨ6, elecampane ℥iii, horehound ℥iii, spikenard ℨ6, white root ℨ6. Boil and pour off to get full strength, strain. Add one pd muscovado sugar, bring to a boil. Throw off the scum, let cool. Add spirits niter, 2 ounces rum or gin ½ pint in hot weather and one gill in cold weather, yet a gill of the best of rum or gin will keep it in all kinds of weather.

For Neuralgia

Tinct nux vomica ℥ij [℥=ounce], strychnine grains ii, sulfate morphea grains ii. Dose: from 5 to 10 drops every six hours, give 10 grains carbonate of iron 3 times a day before eating. This is very good. Try it and I do not think it will fail. B. F. Hale.

---

220 a coastal Mediterranean plant of the lily family

Cholera Med   B, H, 147

Alcohol or brandy 1 quart Opium 1 oz
Sulpher 1 oz Gum Myrrh 1 oz
Cayenne 1 oz Oil Peppermint 20 drops.

xx Kitridge Nerve Ointment
Neats foot oil Spts turpentine
and brandy each 1 gall mix well
and simmer to one gill for Shrunk
cords Rheumatism &c &c .

To prepare Soap   xx
Borax 4 oz Salt 3 oz 2 qts soft water
one gall common soft soap pulverise
the borax and add to the other articles
stir well and and boil 15 minutes
put your cloths in soak over night
wring them out in the morning make a
strong suds put the cloths in boil
well and rence in cold water.

Female Weakness } White pond lilly Solomons seal comfry beth root in wine take freely part of the time and
attention to the syringe and other ablutions part of the time the tansie for ague with Golden this link

Cholera Med. B. F. H.

Alcohol or brandy 1 quart, opium 1 oz, sulfur 1 oz, gum myrrh 1 oz, cayenne 1 oz, oil peppermint 20 drops.

Kitridge Nerve Ointment

Neat's foot oil, spirits turpentine and brandy each 1 gallon, mix well and simmer to one gill. For shrunk cords, rheumatism.

To prepare Soap

Borax 4 oz, salt 5 oz, 2 quarts soft water, one gall common soft soap. Pulverize the borax and add to the other articles, stir well and boil 15 minutes. Put your clothes in, soak over evening, wring them out in the morning, make strong suds, put the clothes in, boil well and rinse in cold water.

Female Weakness

follow the line

White pond lily, Solomon's seal, comfrey, beth root[221] in wine, take freely part of the time and part of the time do tonic for ague with—follow the line – attention to the syringe and other ablutions.

---

221 *Trillium erectum*

96

Salve   X X

Simmer Balm Gilead Buds
Catnip green of Elder to ad
plantain Wormwood Sweet Clover
After boiling strong strain add Mutton
tallow Beeswax white pine turpentine
simmer to a salve of the right
consistance. N B Rosin may be used
instead of the turpentine N B use
cheap Sperits and Water to simmer
the articles in. 1 B tt 7 tt ℔

X X   Rheumatism Tinct
Alcohol 3 pts white helobore ʒj Prickly
ash barries ʒj Black cohush ʒii
Colchicum Seed ʒii Gum Goac ʒv
steep 14 days After shaking filter and
add ʒij Laudanum ʒj Comphry Doce
Commence with a tea spoon full and
increace to what will reet on the stomack
3 or 4 times a day if the stomack is in
a bad condition give my Emitic to
clenze well before giveing the drops

Salve

Simmer Balm Gilead, buds catnip, green of Elder, toad[222], plantain, wormwood, sweet clover. After boiling strong, strain, add mutton tallow, beeswax, white June turpentine, simmer to a salve of the right consistency. N. B. Rosin may be used instead of the turpentine N. B. use cheap spirits and water to simmer the articles in. B. F. Hale

Rheumatism Tinct

Alcohol 3 pints, white hellebore ℥l [℥=ounce], prickly ash berries ℥i, black cohosh ℥ii, colchicum[223] seed ℥ii, gum guaiac ℥v. Steep 14 days after shaking, filter and ℥ij laudanum ℥i comfrey. Dose: commence with a teaspoonful and increase to what will rect on the stomach 3 or 4 times a day, if the stomach is in a bad condition, give my Emetic to cleanse well before giving the drops.

---

222 Eryngium foetidum, toad grass
223 Colchicum Autumnale

xx Kitredge's Ointment

Tobacco one lb — Simmer in chamber lye to get all the strength, press the dregs add one lb hogs lard. Simmer till the urine is taken up then add one oz beeswax 4 oz Rosin one pt Venis terpentine 4 oz oil hemlock 4 oz rectified oil amber incorporate well and it is done, good in all sores piles chaps Salt Rheum tetter Cald Head ℞ ℞ ℞ ℞ ℞ ℞ ℞

For Dysintery xx Dyarrehoea

Bark of the root of high Blackbery ℥j peppermint plant ℥j Black Cerry ℥ij Cinnamon ℥ss Peach meets ℥j Ginger ℥ss Geranium ℥ss Myrrh ℥j Bay Berry ℥ss Nutmegs 2 boil all after being well bruised in watter pour off and mix use sperits to boil it in next use watter put all together strain boil down to one pt and ½ and add ½ pt loaf sugar boil 3 minutes skim when cold add ½ pt french Brandy or Alcohol ℞

Kitridge's Ointment

Tobacco 1 lb. Simmer in urine, chamber lye, to get all the strength. Press the dregs add one lb hogs lard. Simmer till the urine is taken up then add one oz beeswax, 4 oz rosin, one pint Venice turpentine, 4 oz hemlock, 4 oz, rectified oil amber. Incorporate well and it is done. Good in all sores, piles, chaps, salt rheum, tetters, cold head.

For Dysentery Diarrhea

Bark of the root of high blackberry ʒi [ʒ=ounce], peppermint plant ʒi, blackberry ʒii, cinnamon ʒjs, peach meats ʒi, ginger ʒii, geranium ʒjs, myrrh ʒi, bay berry ʒjs, nutmegs 2. Boil all after being well bruised in water, pour off and mix. Use spirits to boil it in, next use water, put all together, strain, boil down to one pint and ½ and add ½ pint loaf sugar. Boil 3 minutes. Skim when cold, add ½ pint French brandy or alcohol.

98   X X   Cement for Cisterns

Ashes sifted 2 parts Clay 2 parts Sand one part mix with oil it will make a Cement as hard as marble impenetratable by water forever & X X ᴙ Godfrey X Cordial ᴙ Tincture of Laudanum 1½ pts Sugar house molasses 2 gall Alcohol 1 qt Water 3 gall & one qt. Carbonate potass 2½ oz oil sassafrass 4 fluid drachms dissolve the potass in the water add the molasses and heat over a gentle fire till they simmer then take off the skum and when cold add the oil sassafrass & Lodanum to the alcohol & then mix all together to use for pain soothing for children used instid of paregoric &   X Wallaces Cough Medicine Raisins ℥iv Elecampane ℥i Bloodroot ℥i Spikenard root ℥iv Digitalis ℥ss Comfrey root ℥iii Hoarhoun ℥i Liquirice stick ℥iii boil all in 2 pts water pour off 3 times strain boil down to one qt add 10 oz Honey & 4 oz loaf sugar boil 3 minutes & skim when partly cold add to every oz & ℥ss best tinct. Lobelia Doce what the stomache will bare without vomiting but

Cement for Cisterns

Ashes sifted 2 parts, clay 3 parts, sand one part, mix with oil. It will make a cement as hard as marble impenetrable by water forever.

Godfrey's Cordial

Tincture of laudanum 1½ pints, sugar house molasses 2 gall, alcohol 1 quart, water 3 gall and 1 quart. Carbonate potash 2½ oz, oil sassafras 4 fluid drachms. Dissolve the potash in the water, add the molasses and heat over a gentle fire till they simmer. Then take off the scum and when cold, add the oil sassafras and laudanum to the alcohol and the mix all together. To use for pain, soothing for children, use instead of paregoric.

Wallace's Cough Medicine

Raisins ℥iv [℥=ounce], elecampane ℥i, bloodroot ℥i, spikenard root ℥iv, digitalis ℥js, comfrey root ℥iii, horehound ℥i, licorice stick ℥iii. Boil all in 2 quarts water, pour off 3 times, strain, boil down to one quart, add 10 oz honey and 4 oz loaf sugar, boil 3 minutes and skim when partly cold, add to every oz and ℥js best tinct lobelia. Dose: what the stomach will bear without vomiting but

in severe cases give enough to cause some
sickness at the Stomach it gives immediate relief—

XX   Quinzy

To prevent its coming on take a tea spoonfull
of salt into the mouth and as it disolves gargle
the throat with it repeat this untill the disease
disapears to discuss the Quinzy in its first
stages make a plaster of hard soap 4 oz sugar
8 oz linsead oil ½ pint rosin 2 oz

Cologne

Oil lavendula ʒi oil lemon ʒij oil
cinnamon viii oil bergamont ʒi oil rosemary ʒijʃ coriphillum gut viii Alcohol
1 pint maschus gutto x mix

XX Affliction of the Spleen

Blue mass 6 grs alloes 2 grs ipicac 1 gr
mix for one doce give a second after which
you will give salts repeat if needed perhaps
cupping will be necessary

XX Remedy called Cureall

1 pt strong spirits wine ʒij Alkenet Root
let this stand two days then add ʒj
camphor and strain through muselin
then add ʒij Opium ʒi-ʒij 2 pts turpen-

in seven cases give enough to cause some sickness at the stomach. It gives immediate relief.

Quinsy[224]

To prevent it coming on, take a teaspoonful of salt into the mouth and as it dissolves, gargle the throat with it. Repeat this until the disease disappears. To discuss the quinsy in its first stages, make a plastic of hard soap 4 oz, sugar 8 oz, linseed oil ½ pint, rosin 2 oz.

Cologne

Oil lavendulan[225] ℥i [℥=ounce], oil lemon ℥ij, oil cinnamon, viii, oil bergamot ℥i, oil rosemary ℥is, caryophyllum[226] gut? viii, alcohol ½ pint, moschus[227], gutta x. Mix.

Affliction of the Spleen

Blue Mass 6 grains, aloes 2 grains, ipecac 1 grain. Mix for one dose, give a second after which you will give salts. Repeat if needed, perhaps cupping will be necessary.

Remedy Called Cure-all

1 pint strong spirits wine, ℥ij [℥=ounce] Alkanet root.[228] Let this stand two days then add ℥i camphor and strain through muslin. Then add ℥ii Opium, ℥i - ℥ij spirits turpentine

---

224 painful pus-filled inflammation or abscess of the tonsils and surrounding tissues
225 Spike Oil
226 Carnation or Clove Pink
227 Musk deer
228 *Alkanna tinctoria* is a member of the borage family with bright blue flowers and a dark red root.

tine it is good for cuts fresh wounds cholic pains in the stomach &c &c for pain in the ear drop it on woll and apply it for internal complaints take 20 or 30 drops on sugar Good Med this is by I.B.H. Male M.D. Rutland Vt.

Ointment for (Calomel ʒj
Tinea Capitis (Prussic Acid m x
or Scall Head. (Solution of Acetate
morphia m x l flowers of Zinc ʒß
Spermactti ʒj mix.

Blistering Plaster № x x
Spanish flys 2 oz Rosin 2 oz Beeswax 2oz
Mutton tallow 2 oz and 2 drachms
Mustard seed 2 drachms Black pepper
2 drachms Viridigriss 1 drachm
Melt the three first articles and when
beginning to boil add the flies &
stir untill cold or well mixed. N B
for winter add 3 oz mutton tallow

Linneament Scierid
3d preppration ʒiv Oreganum ʒj

It is good for cuts, fresh wounds, colic pains in the stomach. For pain in the ear, drop it on wall and apply it for internal complaints. Take 20 or 30 drops on sugar. Good. Med. this is by B. F. Hale M.D. Rutland Vt.

Ointment for Tinea Capitis[229] or Scalp Head Morphea

Calomel ʒi [ʒ=ounce], Prussic Acid[230] mx, Solution of Acetate mxi flowers of zinc ℥ss, spermaceti ʒi. Mix.

Blistering Plaster

Spanish fly 2 oz, rosin 2 oz, beeswax 2 oz, mutton tallow 2 oz and 2 drachms, mustard seed 2 drachms, black pepper 2 drachms, verdigris 1 drachm. Melt the three first articles and when beginning to cool, add the flies. Stir until cold or well mixed. NB
For winter add 3 oz mutton tallow.

Liniment Sacred

3d preparation ℥iv [℥=ounce], Origanum ʒj

---

229 Scalp ringworm
230 also known as hydrocyanic acid or cyanide

Oil Safsafras ℥ss Gum Camphor ℥j Laudanum ℥iv the above for external application for Rheumatism stiffness of the neck from takeing cold stiff joints or any pain wherever situated.

NB how to make the third prepperation Lobelia seed ℥ss Caynne ℥j Myrrh ℥j Nerve root ℥ss or the extract ℥j

℞ Stramonium Ointment — Fresh leaves of Stramonium bruised 5 pounds Lard 14 pounds simmer gently untill the leaves are crisp press out the Lard return to the vessel when cleansed ad'd to every pound of Lard 2 oz of Beeswax melt well together remove from the fire that it may cool and the impurities settle or subside for external inflamations and piles burns and to allay swellings in cows udder.

xx ℞ for Staining Gun Barrels. 1 and ½ oz tinct steal Corrosive Sublimate ½ oz 1½ oz Spts niter 1 oz Blue vitrol 3/4 3 Nitric acid or Aquafortis to be added to 1 qt soft water and one ½ oz Sts nine.

Oil Sassafras ℨjs [ℨ=ounce], gum camphor ℨij, laudanum ℨiv. The above for external application for rheumatism, stiffness of the neck from taking cold, stiff joints or any pain wherever situated. NB How to make the third preparation: lobelia seed ℨjs, cayenne ℨj, myrrh ℨj, nerve root ℨjs or the extract ℨj.

Stramonium Ointment

Fresh leaves of stramonium bruised 5 pounds, lard 14 pounds. Simmer gently until the leaves are crisp, press out the lard. Return to the vessel when cleansed. Add to every pound of lard 2 oz of beeswax, melt well together, remove from the fire that it may cool, and the impurities settle or subside. For external inflammations and piles, burns, and to allay swellings in cow's udder.

Rx for Staining Gun Barrels

1½ oz tinct steel, corrosive sublimate ½ oz, 1½ oz spirits niter, 1 oz blue vitriol, ¾ oz nitric acid or aqua fortis to be added to 1 quart soft water and 1½ oz spirits wine.

102

xx To case harden by S.A.P. Hale
Prusiate Potashe 2 oz Oxalic Acid
1 oz. Zovil

xx Emory for inside of Barrels
Emorine, this is the name of the preperaton
Block tin 7 parts Antimony 1 part
lead 4 parts good,

xxx Antiphlogistic & Cooling Plaster
Red lead ℥j & good vinegar ½ pint Sweet oil
½ pt gum camphor ℥j one oz made fine put the
lead vinegar & oil togather in an earthan pot
set the pot into a kettle of coals & boil it untill the vinegar is evaporated then add the
camphor & boil it down to the consistance
of wax then take it out and work like wax
the above must be stired constantly while over
the fire it is good for inflamations sore canker
lumps & ague in the breast —

xx Indian Salve. Equil parts hard
soap, Rosin Brown Sugar. linseed oil
to be well mixed over @ slow fire and if
to soft add more Rosin for all kinds of

To Case Harden by S. A. J. Hale

Prussiate of Potash[231] 2 oz, Oxalic Acid 1 oz. Good.

Emory for Inside of Barrels

Emorine, this is the name of the preparation. Block tin 7 parts, Antimony 1 part, lead 4 parts. Good.

Antiphlogistic or Cooling Plaster

Red lead ℥iv [℥=ounce], good vinegar ½ pint, sweet oil ½ pint, gum camphor one oz, made fine, put the lead, vinegar, and oil together in an earthen pot. Set the pot into a kettle of coals and boil it until the vinegar is evaporated, then add the camphor and boil it down to the consistency of wax. Then take it out and work like wax. The above must be stirred constantly while over the fire, it is good for inflammations, sore canker, lumps, and ague in the breast.

Indian Salve

Equal parts hard soap, rosin, brown sugar, linseed oil. To be will mixed over a slow fire, and if too soft, add more rosin. For all kinds of

---

231 potassium ferrocyanide

ulcers tightness of the breast for sore
throat quinzy apply to the throat. Good,
For Ague and

Fever ×× ⎰ Peach meats or Pits, 2 oz
Flunalbus & tinis ⎱ to a pint of best Brandy
kept warm for one week dose, a tea
spunful 3 or 4 times a day if the habbit is
cold add a little Cayne or Myrrh.

Composition ⎱ Plurisy root 1 lb Bayberry
×× Improved ⎰ Bark of the root 1 lb Sass-
the dose in a tea spoon-
full in sweetening water   afras bark 4 oz Cholic Root
every ½ hour
4 oz Ginger 1 lb Clives 2 oz Cayne 2 oz
Dose as of the former composition a
good Diaphoretic or sweating powder.
×× Alterative. B.#.'Hab Goac wood 2 lbs
Pipsisawa 1 and ½ pds Burdock sead
and root 1 and ½ pd Yellow Parrilla
and Sassaprille 1 lb Blue cohush ½ pd
Steep in hot water over night slow boil
one hour strain add more water let stand
in a hot place 3 or 4 hours boil an hour
and strain so proceed as above until
the strength is all extracted strain all and
reduce to 16 qts add 2 gallons sugar

ulcers, tightness of the breast. For sore throat, quinsy, apply to the throat.

For Ague and Fever—Fluor albus and tonic

Peach meats or pits 2 oz, to a pint of best brandy kept warm for 1 week. Dose, a teaspoonful 3 or 4 times a day. If the hobbit? is cold add a little cayenne or myrrh.

Composition Improved

Pleurisy root 1 lb, bayberry bark of the root 1 lb, sassafras bark 4 oz, cholic root[232] 1 lb, cloves 2 oz, cayenne 2 oz. Dose as of the former composition a good diaphoretic sweating preventer.

Alternative

Guaiac wood 2 lbs, pipsissewa[233] 1½ pds, burdock seed and root 1½ pd, yellow perilla[234] and sarsaparilla 1 lb, blue cohosh ½ pd. Steep in hot water over night. Slow boil one hour, strain, add more water, let stand in a hot place 3 or 4 hours, boil an hour and strain. So proceed as above until the strength is all extracted, strain all and reduce to 16 quarts. Add 2 gallons sugar

---

232 Aletris farinosa
233 chimaphila umbellate, a wintergreen
234 a mint

104

house or other good molasses added
2 qts best gin essence Sassafras 2 oz
Dose a wine glass full 3 times a day....

Liver Syrup B W⟨?⟩ + Hale
Blue flag root ½ pds Sassaprilla 5 pds
Guaiacum shavings 2 lbs Sassafras
bark 1½ pds Elder flowers 1 lb Blood
root 4 oz Licquorice 1 lb Elecampane
1 lb Black Cherry bark 1 lb Spikenard Root
1 lb Mountain Liver wort 2 lbs bittersweet
bark of the root if it can be got 1 lb put
all in 8 qts cheap spirits and water
sufficient to a little more than to cover
the articles boil in a tinned copper vessel
and pour off and repeatedly boil and
pour off untill the full strength is
obtained strain the whole let stand
to settle pour off and boil down to
4 galls and add 25 pds clarified
Sugar boil a few minutes and let
Stand 24 hours to settle Dose a wine
glass 3 or 4 times a day add to th above
4 oz carraway seed. (this is good)

house or other good molasses and 2 quarts best gin, essence sassafras 2 oz. Dose: a wine glass full 3 times a day.

Liver Syrup B. F. Hale

Blue Flag 1½ pds, sarsaparilla 5 pds, Guaiacum shaving 2 lbs, sassafras bark 1½ pds, elder flowers 1 lb, bloodroot 4 oz, licorice 1 lb, elecampane 1 lb, black cherry bark 1 lb, spikenard root 1 lb, mountain liver wort 2 lbs, bittersweet bark of the root if it can be got 1 lb. Put all in 8 quarts cheap spirits and water sufficient to a little more than to cover the articles. Boil in a tinned copper vessel and pour off, and repeatedly boil and pour off until the full strength is obtained. Strain the whole, let stand to settle, pour off and boil down to 4 gall and add 25 pints clarified sugar, boil a few minutes, and let stand 24 hours to settle. Dose: a wine glass 3 or 4 times a day. Add to the above 4 oz caraway seed. This is good.

Horse and Man Linneament

xx

one half pt Spirits turpentine the same quantity tanners oil 2 oz Sugar lead 2 oz Salt peter 2 oz Oil vitrol. pulverise the lead and salt peter add the two first articles and when well shook together add to oil vitrol leaving the vessel open for a little time then close it for fever sores and all ill conditioned old sores sores on horses as galling of the saddle, harness &c &c.

x Diptheria 2 Freely swob the back of the mouth & throat with a wash made of table salt 2 drachms black pepper golden seal nitrate potash allum 1 drachm mix & pulverise put into a teacup filled half full of boiling water stir well and fill the cup with good vinegar – use every half hour one two or four hours as recovery progresses – the patient should swallow a little each time – to the outside apply the following spts turpentine sweet oil aqua ammonia mixed well bathe the whole of the throat and to the breast bone every 3 or 4 hours keep flannel on the parts &c of the time — Good – better – best – first

Horse and Man Liniment

One half pint spirits turpentine, the same quantity tanner's oil, ℥js [℥=ounce] sugar lead, ℥js saltpeter, ℥js oil vitriol. Pulverize the lead and saltpeter. Add the first two articles and when well shaken together add the oil vitriol, leaving the vessel open for a little time, then close it. For fever sores on horses as galling of the saddle, harness.

Diphtheria

Freely swab the back of the mouth and throat with a wash made of table salt 8 drachms, black pepper, golden seal, nitrate potash, alum 1 drachm. Mix and pulverize. Put into a teacup filled half full of boiling water, stir well and fill the cup with good vinegar. Use every half hour, one, two or four hours as recovery progresses. The patient should swallow a little each time. To the outside, apply the following: spirits turpentine, sweet oil, aqua ammonia, mixed well. Bathe the whole of the throat and to the breast bone every 3 or four hours. Keep flannel on the part all the time. Good. Better. Best. First Rate.

106

× Last- Alterative

Garget or poke root — 1 lb gaac wood 6 oz
Sassafras bark 6 oz to make 4 qts syrup put all
in water make steaming hot and keep it so
for 12 hours then boil one hour or two and
press out the fluid next add spirits enough to
cover it let stand a number of days to get the
strength or put it in a percolating machine &
run over & over to get the full strength & press all
the tincture out and add a pound of sugar to
every qt of the tea & tincture And bring to a boil
skim cool & bottle

Hair Dye
Lac Sulphor 4 oz Sugar lead 4 oz
one pint bay rum ½ pint jamacia rum tincture
Lobelia 1 oz 1 qt rain water 1 table spoon full
Salt

Another } Sugar of lead 1 oz   Cristalised nitrate silver 10 grs
                                 spts ammonia 1½ ʒs
         Lac Sulphor ½ ʒ
         Rose Water   1 gill
Rain water } Coperas   1 qt
                                           1 drachm
Rain water 1 qt

× Strengthening Plaster
Rosin 2 lb beeswax 1½ lb bergundy pitch ½ lb
melt all together over a slow fire when warm but no

Last Alterative

Garget or poke root 1 lb, guaiac wood 6 oz, sassafras bark 6 oz. To make 4 quarts syrup put all in water, make steaming hot and keep it so for 12 hours, then boil one hour or two and press out the fluid. Next add spirits, enough to cover it. Let stand a number of days to get the strength or put it in a percolating machine and run over and over to get the full strength. I press all the tincture out and add a pound of sugar to every quart of the tea and tincture and bring to a boil. Cool and bottle.

Hair Dye

Lae? sulfur 4 oz, sugar lead 4 oz, one pint bay rum, ½ pint Jamaican rum, tincture lobelia 1 oz, 1 quart rain water, 1 tablespoonful salt.

Another

Sugar lead 1 oz, Lae? sulfur ½ oz, rose water and copperas, crystallized nitrate silver 10 grains, 2 pints ammonia 1½ ʒ
[ʒ=ounce]
Rain water 1 quart

Strengthening Plaster

Rosin 2 lb, beeswax 1½ lb, burgundy pitch ½ lb. Melt all together over a slow fire when warm, but not so as to burn, add one lb balsam fir, stir well together (perfectly) and try a little in cold water and if to hard add more balsam & if to soft add a little more rosin when right work it as you would shoemakers wax said to be excellent —

Rheumatism ₂ Cohash 4 oz black cohush 3 oz prickley ash berries 2 oz bloodroot 2 oz alcohol 3 pints poke berries 4 oz swamp sassafras 1 oz

Last Alterative. B. V. Wav
Saksaprillia 4 oz Sasafras bark 2 oz Guac wood 2 oz one qt whisky one of Alcohol first added. Iris Irisversicolor 2 oz poke or garget 4 oz Yellow dock root 3 oz Burdock root green 4 oz Mandrake root 1 oz Senna 2½ oz Elder flowers 2 oz Bittersweet 2 oz. Keep warm one day run off dry press boil over and over to get all strength boil down and with the spirit run have 3 qts add 1 lb Sugar to the qt and lastly add the spent run cool settle and run off for use the above weights 1 lb and ½ oz and ½ in a dry state before steeping

so as to burn, add one lb balsam fir. Stir well together (perfectly) and try a little in cold water, and if too hard, add more balsam and if too soft add a little more rosin. When right, work it as would shoemaker's wax. Said to be excellent.

Last Alterative

Sarsaparilla 4 oz, sassafras bark 2 oz, Guaiac wood 2 oz, one quart whiskey, one of alcohol, first added. Iris versicolor 2 oz, poke or garget 4 oz, yellow dock root 1 oz, senna 2½ oz, elder flowers 2 oz, bittersweet 2 oz. Keep warm one day, run off, dry, press, boil over and over to get all the strength, boil down and with the sperit run(?) have 5 quarts, add 1 lb sugar to the quart and lastly add the sperit run. Cool, settle, and pour off for use. The above weighs 1 lb and 11 oz and ½ in a dry state before steeping.

108

Chronic Rheumatism
× ×

Prickly ash berrys 4 oz Poke root or ganger 4 oz Black cohush Root 8 oz Alcohol 4 pts water 1 and ½ pts grind the roots and tinct 14 days filter and add the tinct. Tinct of white swamp helibore 8 oz Tinct Guaiacum 4 oz shake well together and commence with 1 tea spoonful every 3 hours and increas the doce to all the head and stomach will bear take the bead after soaking the feet and give sudorific drinks every fiew minutes and every 2 or 3 hours, the drops as above directed avoice every cause of fever and repeat every 24 hours the same opperation produce a free sweating every 24 hours NB the next recpt is to make the Sudorific drops used with this medicine.

Sudorific Drops × ×

Ipicac 2 oz
Saffron 2 oz
Virginia snake Root 2 oz
Opium 2 oz
Holland gin or good Rum or Alcohol 3 qts at ⅌ pret let stand 2 weeks and filter often agitating the tinct.

Chronic Rheumatism

Prickly ash berries 4 oz, poke root or garget 4 oz, black cohosh root 8 oz, alcohol 4 pints, water 1½ pints. Grind the roots and tinct 14 days, filter and add the tinct. Tinct of white swamp hellebore 8 oz, tinct guaiacum[235] 4 oz. Shake well together and commence with 1 teaspoonful every 3 hours and increase the dose to all the head and stomach will bear. Take the bead? after soaking the feet and give sudorific drinks every few minutes and every 2 or 3 hours. The drops as above directed, avoid every cause of fever, and repeat every 24 hours the same operation produce a free sweating every 24 hours. NB. The next step is to make the Sudorific drops used with this medicine.

Sudorific Drops

Spicae[236] 2 oz
Saffron 2 oz
Virginia snake root[237] 2 oz
Opium 2 oz
Holland gin or good rum or alcohol 3 quarts at 76 pct, let stand 2 weeks and filter, often agitating the tinct.

---

235 An ornamental evergreen tree with pretty rich blue flowers
236 Spike lavender essential oil
237 *Aristolochia serpentiaria*

Injection for Gonorrhoea

White vitrol	1 drachm
Sugar lead	1 "
Chloride of Soda	½ "
Loaf Sugar	1 "
Pulverised Alumn	½ "
Rosa Flora	1 "
Pure water	1.6 oz

Sulphate Zinc 1 Drachm

simmer all over a slow fire 15 minutes, when cool strain and put in well corked bottles.

Vegitable Salve

1 pd lard ½ pd rosin 10 oz elder bark boil over a slow fire 30 minutes strain put in small boxes for sale use for all cuts sores old sores and every case where a salve is needed. Good & Liver Lungs and Blood. R℟ ℞

Poke or Sargit Root 4 oz Mandrake root 4 oz Blue flag root 4 oz black root or Culver Root 4 oz Blood Root 4 oz Safsapirel 8 oz Yellow dock root 8 oz Goose wort 4 oz Safsofrafs Bark 4 oz Ellecampane Root 4 oz

Injection for Gonorrhea

White vitriol	1 drachm
Sugar Lead	1 drachm
Chloride of Soda	½ drachm
Loaf Sugar	1 drachm
Pulverized Alum	½ drachm
Rosa Flora	1 drachm
Pure water	16 oz
Sulfate Zinc	1 drachm

Simmer all over a slow fire 15 minutes, when cool, strain and put in well-corked bottle.

Vegetable Slave

1 pd lard, ½ pd rosin, 10 oz elder bark. Boil over a slow fire 30 minutes, strain, put in small boxes for sale. Use for all cuts, sores, old sores, and every ease where a salve is needed. Good

Liver, Lungs and Blood B. F. Hale

Poke or garget root 4 oz, mandrake root 4 oz, blue flag root 4 oz, black root or Culver root 4 oz, bloodroot 4 oz, sarsaparilla 8 oz, yellow dock root 8 oz, Guaiac wood 4 oz, sassafras bark 4 oz, elecampane root 4 oz

Stillingia Root 4 oz Slipery Elm 4 oz Prickly ash 2 oz Pipsisiwa 4 oz prepare as for syrup Sasaparilla adding 12 oz sugar to every pt— add to the above tag alder Bark 4 oz chery Bark 4 oz. Good

xx A great Linneament for Scrofula Inflamation Chronic Rheumatism wounds on man or beast scalds sprains Bruises contractions of cords sinews and to be applyed to the palpebra muscles of the eyes when there is inflamed or sore eyes. Oil Origanum 1 lb Oil Rosemary 1 lb Olive or Sweet oil 2 lbs tinct Spanish flies ½ lb Spts turpentine ½ lb strongest spts Camphor 1 oz mix all well together for the above uses NB. be sure that the Origanum and Rosemary are pure. Good

x Chery Pectoral. Sulphate Morphine 4 grs Tinct Blood Root 2 drachms wine of antimony and wine of Ipicac each 3 drachms Syrup of wild chery 3 oz mix an active expectorant to be used in a distressing and unceasing cough good in many kinds of coughs. Good

Stillingia root[238] 4 oz, slippery elm 4 oz, prickly ash 2 oz, Pipsissewa [239] 4 oz. Prepare as for syrup sarsaparilla adding 12 oz sugar to every pint—add to the above tag alder[240] bark 4 oz, cherry bark 4 oz. Good.

A Great Liniment for Scrofula, Inflammation, Chronic Rheumatism, Wounds on Man or Beast, Scalds, Sprains, Bruises, Contractions of Cords, Sinews, and to be applied to the palpebra muscles of the eyes when there is inflamed or sore eyes.

Oil Origanum 1 lb, oil rosemary 1 lb, olive or sweet oil 2 lbs, tinct Spanish flies ½ lb, turpentine ½ lb, strongest spirits camphor 1 oz. Mix all well together for the above cases NB. Be sure that the Origanum and Rosemary are pure. Good.

Cherry Pectoral Sulfate

Morphine 4 grains, bloodroot 2 drachms, wine of antimony and wine of Ipecac each 3 drachms, syrup of wild cherry 3 oz. Mix. An active expectorant to be used in a distressing and unceasing cough. Good in many kinds of cough. Good.

---

238 Stillingia is a perennial herb in the spurge family
239 bitter wintergreen
240 best guess, tag alder is a shrub used in medicine

R for making vegitable oil to burn in lamps Suppherior to Oil or gas or common burning fluid to one gall of 90 to 95 pres- of Alcohol add one qt of Rectified spts turpentine or as much as the Alcohol will cut and become transpasent by shaking theme well together in a bottle to the above add ¼ oz Oil Rosemary then the article extinguish the lights when you fill the lamp keep the vessel containing the oil well stopen PS if the oil of Rosemary is to highly Rectified to give it the desired collor add a little tinct Carcuma— preperations on a small scale for the above. make some ⟨For 2 qts Comp'd Syrup Sarsapirilla for the blood Syphlis Scrofula and all Imphurities of the circulating fluid Bitter sweet 2 oz Yellow dock root 8 oz Ipsisiwa top & root 2 oz sarsa- purilla root 4 oz Guac wood 8 oz Sassafras bark 2 & 3 oz Elder flowers 2 oz mandrake root 1½ oz blue flag Root 2 oz put all in water boil slowly pour of twice then put in the percolato

Rx for making vegetable oil to burn in lamps, superior to oil or gas or common burn fluid:

To one gallon of 90 to 95 proof of alcohol add one quart of rectified spirits turpentine or as much as the alcohol will cut and become transparent by shaking them well together in a bottle. To the above add ¼ oz oil rosemary, then the article extinguish the light. When you fill the lamp, keep the vessel containing the oil well stopped. PS, if the oil of rosemary is too highly rectified to give it the desired color, add a little tinct curcuma. Preparations on a small seal for the above.

Syrup Sarsaparilla

For 2 quarts, Confit for the blood, Syphilis, Scrofula, and all Impurities of the calculating fluid. Bittersweet 2 oz, yellow dock root 8 oz, Pipsissewa top and root 2 oz, sarsaparilla root 4 oz, Guaiac wood 3 oz, sassafras bark 2½ oz, elder flowers 2 oz, mandrake root 1½ oz, blue flag root 2 oz. Put all in water, boil slowly, for of twice then put in the percolator.

112

add Spirits 1 pt or rum of one pint set by and boil all the decoction down to 3 pints & ad one lb refined sugar to each pint of the syrup 1 oz hydridate potassa to be added to each qt of syrup. Dose from a third to half a wine glass 3 or 4 times a day. After running through the alcohol or spirits you will put through hot water to obtain all the strength and add to the first decoction before boiling down to 3 pints and procede as above directed.

+ To Produce Salivation
Equal parts finely pulverised Mandrake root Blue flag root & prickly ash bark mixed together & given in 6 to 8 times in the course of 24 hours 2 in a day or two salivate copiously if they are this effect will not be produced if they are allowed to have a purgative action

+ Gonorrhoea

Spirits nitre	4 oz	
Balsom fir	2 oz	Dose a teaspoonfull
Sweet or almond oil	3 oz	3 times a day
Gum Camphor	℈ ij	
Solution Gum Arabic	4 oz	
Laudanum	2 oz	Mix

Add spirits 1 pint or rum of one pint. Set by and boil all of the decoction down to 8 pints and add one lb refined sugar to each pint of the syrup, 1 oz hydrate potash to be added to each quart of syrup. Dose: From a third to half a wine glass 3 or 4 times a day. After running through the alcohol or spirits, you will put through hot water to obtain all of the strength and add to the first decoction before boiling down to 3 pints and proceed as above directed.

To Reduce Salination

Equal parts finely pulverized mandrake root, blue flag root and prickly ash bark mixed together and give in 6 to 8 times in the course of 24 hours, and in a day or two salivate copiously. This effect will not be produced if they are allowed to have a purgative action.

Gonorrhea

Spirits nitre 4 oz
Balsam fir 2 oz
Sweet or almond oil 3 oz
Gum camphor Ӡij
Solution gum Arabic 4 oz
Laudanum 2 oz
Mix. Dose: a teaspoonful 3 times a day.

For Lungs & Liver

Blood root	12 oz	Wild indigo	4 oz
Cherry bark	8 "	Tamarack bark	6 "
Anise seed	12 "	Elecampane root	6 "
Black Cohosh root	12 "	Sassafras bark	10 "
Digitalis herb	6 "	Mandrake root	8 "
Squills	4 "	Blue flag root	8 "
Elder flowers	8 "	Spikenard root	8 "
Comfrey root	4 "	Smart weed	8 "
White root	10 "	Scull cap herb	8 "
Bugle weed	8 "	Hour houn herb	6 "
Cocash root	8 "	Valerian root	8 "
Golden seal root	4 "	Skunk cabbage root	8 "
Liquorice stick	6 "	Seneca snake root	4 "
Bitter root	6 "	Culver root	6 "
		Peach leaves or pits	10 "
		Yellow dock root	8 "

Dandelion 8 oz

N B there must be 6 gallons & 1 qt of spirits used
½ proof alcohol

First wet the articles with warm water let stand 24 hours transfer to the perculator & add spirits enough to run off 2 gallons after remaining on the roots 12 hours before turning the fossel for a discharge set the 2 galons by by its self add the other spirit by degrees & run it all through & a part the second time or even the third time next add hot water by degrees

For Lungs and Liver

Bloodroot 12 oz	Wild indigo 4 oz	
Cherry bark 8 oz	Tamarack bark 6 oz	
Anise seed 12 oz	Elecampane root 6 oz	
Black cohosh root 12 oz	Sassafras bark 10 oz	
Digitalis herb 6 oz	Mandrake root 8 oz	
Squills 4 oz	Blue Flag root 8 oz	
Elder flowers 8 oz	Spikenard root 8 oz	
Comfrey root 4 oz	Smart weed 8 oz	
White root 10 oz	Skull cap herb 8 oz	
Bugle weed 8 oz	Horehound herb 5 oz	
Cocash root 6 oz	Valerian root 8 oz	
Golden seal root 4 oz	Skunk cabbage root 8 oz	
Licorice stick 6 oz	Seneca snake root 4 oz	
Bitterroot 6 oz	Culver root 6 oz	
Peach leaves or pits 10 oz	Yellow dock root 8 oz	
Dandelion 6 oz		

NB there must be 6 gallons & 1 gal of spirits used 76 percent alcohol

First, wet the articles with warm water, let stand 24 hours, transfer to the percolator, and add spirits enough to run off 2 gallons after remaining in the roots 12 hours. Before turning the vessel for a discharge, set the 2 gallons by itself, add the other spirit by degrees and run it all through and part the second time or even the third time. Next add hot water by degrees

114

and run off till the liquor passes of nearly tasteless & boil it down untill the percoulated shirit & water will make nine gallons — settle filter if needed & add 54 lbs crushed sugar bring to a boil throw off the scum as it rises & lastly cool & to every pint add 12 grs emetic tarter & 2 drachms laudanum & 8 drops prugic acid — instad of using sugar for the above may use as many pounds of golden syrup (that is) the molasses called golden syrup at the store the spirit used for the above should be 4th proof or a little higher, perhaps 76 percel — not higher

{ Diarrhoea } Blackberry rut — 2 oz
　　　　　　Geranium 2 g
　　　　　Burnt Rhuebarb 1 oz
　　　One large nutmeg
　　　　Cinnamon 2 drachms
make fine put in a qt water steep and pour off 3 times simmute one qt add 1 pt best brandy 1 lb loaf sugar one oz No 6 one oz parrigoric Dose according to age and circumstances move the bowels with Rhubarb and Saleratus before giving giving the above.

and run off till the liquor passes of nearly tasteless? and boil it down until the percolator spirit and water will make nine gallons—settle, filter if needed, and add 54 lbs crushed sugar, bring to a boil. Throw off the scum as it rises and lastly cool and to every pint add 12 grains emetic tartar and 2 drachms laudanum and 8 drops prussic acid[241]. Instead of using sugar for the above med, use as many pounds of golden syrup, that is the molasses called golden syrup at the store, the spirit used for the above should be 4th proof or a little higher, perhaps 76 percent, not higher.

Diarrhea

Blackberry root 2 oz
Geranium 2 oz
Burnt Rhubarb 1 oz
One large nutmeg
Cinnamon 2 drachms
Make fine, put in a quart water, steep, and pour off 3 times, simmer to 1 quart, add 1 pint best brandy, 1 lb loaf sugar, one oz No. 6, one oz paregoric. Dose according to age and circumstances move the bowels with rhubarb and saleratus before giving the above.

---

241 Hydrocyanic acid or cyanide, a lethal toxin

& Lucys ague pills

Put in 3 and ½ pints of good brandy or
other good spirits one oz Golden seal
Pulverized half oz good Composition
half oz Bloodroot Dose all the stomach
will bear 3 or 4 times a day

(Hydro Alcoholic) Take coursely powered
Ext Blue cohosh) Blue cohosh Root 2 lb
Alcohol sufficient quantity moisten the cohosh
with 2 pts Alcohol let stand 24 hours then
transfer it to a displacement apparatus and
gradualy add Alcohol untill it passes off without
tast of the root distill off the greater part
of the Alcohol from the liquor after filtering
it and evaporate the residue to a propper
consistance to the powder in the displacement apparatus add gradualy sufficient quantity of water untill the liquor passes but slightly impregnated with the properties of the
cohosh heat the filtered liquor to the boiling
point strain evaporate to the propper consisten-
cix, mix the Alcohol and aqueous ext while each
are hot and each are cold. B.H. Mar MD

Lucy's Ague Bitters

Put in 3 ½ pints of good brandy or other good spirits one oz Golden seal pulverized, half oz good Composition, half oz Bloodroot. Dose, all the stomach will bear 3 or 4 times a day.

Hydro Alcoholic Ext Blue Cohosh

Take coarsely powdered blue cohosh root 2 lb, alcohol sufficient quantity moisten the cohosh with 2 pints alcohol, let stand 24 hours, then transfer it to a displacement apparatus and gradually add alcohol until it passes of without cast of the root. Distill off the greater part of the alcohol from the liquor after filtering it and evaporate the residue to a proper consistency to the powder in the displacement apparatus. Add gradually sufficient quantity of water until the liquor passes, but slightly impregnated with the properties of the whish. Heat in filtered liquor to the boiling point, strain, evaporate to the proper consistency mix. Mix the alcohol and aqueous extract while each one hot and each one cold.
B. F. Hale MD

116

+ Vegitable Drops.

To cure corns, warts, Moles tetters Ringworm and toothache can be removed in three minutes free of charge and without pain Pole evels, fistula wind galls on horses or any morbid or any morbid growth on beasts cured in one application. For warts Pair thin put on one drop of the salve leave it on 3 minutes wash it off press it out and oil it Corns must not be paired because now moles the same they will fall off like a scale in two days now tetter or ringworm make a solution by adding 4 times the quality of soft water that you do of the salve apply it leave on 5 minutes then wash it all clean and oil it with sweet oil now the tooth ache put a little in the the tooth on cotton leave it in 3 minutes take it out and rinse the mouth with vineagr it will never ache again. Pole evel saturate some cotton with the salve place it in the hole 10 minutes then wash it oil it and bandage with oiled rag, Fistula the same as Pole evel The Reciept now

direction on next page

Vegetable Drops

To cure corns, warts, moles, tetters, ringworm, and toothache. Can be removed in three minutes free of charge and without pain. Poll evils, fistula wind galls on horses or and morbid growth on beasts cured in one application. For warts: pare thin, put on one drop of the salve, leave it on 3 minutes, wash it off, press it out and oil it. Corns must not be pared, be careful. Now moles, the same, they will fall off like a scab in two days, Now tetters or ringworm make a solution by adding 4 times the quantity of soft water that you do of the salve, apply it, leave it on 5 minutes then wash it all clean and oil it with sweet oil. Now the toothache, put a little in the tooth on cotton, leave it in three minutes, take it out and rinse the mouth with vinegar; it will never ache again. Poll evil, saturate some cotton with the salve, place it in the hole 10 minutes, then wash it, oil it and bandage with oiled rages. Fistula, the same as poll evil. The recipe now the first on next page.

Caustic Potassa 1 lb Water 1½ pts
Mix let stand 4 hours to digest — and
add 1 oz pulverised borax fill your
bottle most full and fill them up
with florn cork with cotton and bind
over with bladder this is Infalible, B.W.W

Mrs Wallace A W Take Lobelia leaf & seed blood root
Comp Tinc) Skunk cabbage root asarabacca or
Lobelia 7 (wild ginger root Pleurisy root
each coarsely powdered 1 oz water or vinegar 1
pint — Alcohol 8 pts Macerate 14 days & filter
through paper good emetics for Children & infants
safely used in croup whooping cough Bronchitis
Asthma convulsions & in all cases where an emetic
is required to be used as an expectorant
pleuritic affections wherever expectorants are
indicated in grown folks. for an expectorant
1 to 2 two tea spoonfulls in slipery elm tea from
3 to 5 times per day Kep the stomache & bowel
regular in all cases §X Syrup of wild cherry — Macerate
4 oz of the powdered bark in 12 fluid ozs of water for 2 days
put it in a perculator & run the infusion through till it
comes clear perhaps add more water till you obtain 12 fluid
ozs of the infusion disolve 12 oz of loaf sugar Doce ½ to 1 oz
3 times a day

Caustic potash 1 lb, water 1½ pints, Mix, let stand 4 hours to digest and add 1 oz pulverized borax. Fill your bottle most full and fill them up with flour. Cork with cotton and bind over with bladder. This is infallible. B. F. H. Mr. Wallace A. H.

Comp Tinc Lobelia

Skunk cabbage root, asarum canadense[242] or wild ginger root, pleurisy root[243], each coarsely powdered 1 oz, water, or vinegar 1 pint, alcohol 3 pints macerate 14 days and filter through paper. Good emetics for children and infants, safely used in croups, whooping cough, bronchitis, asthma, convulsions and in all cases when an emetic is required to be used as an expectorant. Pleuritic affections where expectorants are indicated in grown folks for an expectorant 1 to 2 teaspoonfuls in slippery elm tea from 3 to 5 times a day. Rub the stomach and bowels regularly in all cases

Syrup of Wild Cherry

Macerate 4 oz of the powdered bark in 12 fluid oz of water for 2 days, put it in a percolator and run the infusion through till it comes clear, perhaps add more water till you obtain 12 fluid ozs of the infusion, dissolve 13 oz of loaf sugar. Dose ½ to 1 oz 3 times a day.

---

242 Wild ginger, *Asarum canadense*, is unrelated to commercially available ginger; however, it is named wild ginger because of the similar taste and smell of the roots.
243 A brilliant orange flowered herb

118

Comp ~~tinct~~ Syrup of Rhubarb
Neutralizing cordial 113, 44, 441

Take of India Rhei in corse powder and pure carbonate of Potassa each 2 oz golden seal Cinnamon each 1 oz refined sugar 4 lbs brandy 1 gall oil Peppermint 20 drops macerate the Rheubarb Golden seal and cinnamon in ½ gall Brandy 6 hours with a gentle heat — next put the mass in a vessel with fine holes in a tin bottom add the other 2 qts of Brandy let it pass off add water till the whole strength is obtained or the liquor comes off tasteless to this add the carbonate Potassa sugar and oils Peppermint the Peppermint being rubbed up and well mixed with the sugar to absorb it and mix the liquors well together shake well Alcohol at 76 proof instead of Brandy good in obstinate constipation acidity of the Stomach Dyspepsia, and as a laxative in pregnancy and where piles are present for Diarrhoea Dysentary cholera morbus Cholera infantum and in the same Doses as the composition powders

Comp Syrup of Rhubarb
Neutralizing Cordial B. F. H.

Take of India Rhubarb in coarse powder and pure carbonate of potash each 2 oz, golden seal, cinnamon each 1 oz, refined sugar 4 lbs, brandy 1 gallon, oil peppermint 20 drops, macerate the rhubarb, golden seal, and cinnamon in ½ gallon brandy 6 hours with a gentle heat. Next put the mass in a vessel with fine holes in a tin bottom, add the other 2 quarts of brandy. Let it pass off, add water till the whole strength is obtained or the liquor comes off tasteless. To this add the carbonate potash, sugar and oils peppermint, the peppermint being rubbed up and well mixed with the sugar to absorb it and mix the liquors well together. Shake well. Alcohol at 76 percent instead of brandy. Good on obstinate constipation especially of the stomach, dyspepsia, and as a laxative in pregnancy and where piles are present.
For diarrhea, dysentery, cholera morbus, cholera infantum and in the same diseases as the composition powders.

of Rhuebarb Doce for an adult a table spoonfull every hour or two according to the urgency of the case

Indian Linneament — ℞ ℣ ⁊ ⁋
Externaly for Rheumatism Tics Dolorroux Rickets ague in the face and breast quinsey pain in the side and breast plurisy pain in decayed teeth nervous spasms chilblanes swellings of all kinds pain in joints white swellings lumbago internaly from 5 to 6 drops with distress inwardly.

Oil Wormwood	℥j
" Sassafras	℥ij
" Hemlock	℥j
" Red Ceadar	℥j
" Terpentine	℥j
" Cayune	℥j
" Oreganum	℥j
" Peppermint	℥ij
" Spearmint	℥ij
Tinct Nux vomica	℥ij
" Swamp helibor	℥ij
Spts Beladonna	℥ss
Laudanum	℥iii

Camphor ℥j

of rhubarb. Dose for an adult a tablespoonful every hour or two according to the urgency of the case.

Indian Liniment B.F.H.

Externally for rheumatism, Tic douloureux[244], rickets, ague in the face and breast, quinsy, pain in the side and breast, pleurisy, pain in decayed teeth, nervous spasms, chilblains, swellings of a kinds, pain in joints, white swellings, lumbago, internally from 5 to 60 drops with distress inwardly.

Oil wormwood ℥j [℥=ounce]
Oil sassafras ℥ij
Oil hemlock ℥j
Oil Red Cedar ℥j
Oil Turpentine ℥j
Oil Cayenne ℥j
Oil Origanum ℥j
Oil Peppermint ℥ij
Oil Spearmint ℥ij
Tinct Nux Vomica ℥ij
Tinct Swamp Hellebore ℥ij
Spirits Belladonna ℥js
Laudanum ℥iii
Camphor ℥ij

---

244 a severe, stabbing pain to one side of the face.

X Elder Berry Wine

Pull the berries from the stalks & put them in a tub pour boiling water on them 2 gallons water to 8 gallons of berries press them down into the liquor & cover closely let remain in 24 hours press the juice from the berries clean as possible and to every gallon of this juice add 3 lbs of sugar 1 oz of cloves 1 oz ginger boil 20 minutes skim thoroughly while still hot put it into a cask or stone jug or bottles fill the jug or cask full add to every gall one spoonful of new yeast and stir it well together with a stick fresh berries and picked in a dry day is best —

X Good Black Ink

    Prucciate Potass   24 grs
    bicornate potass   12 grs
    Extract logwood   1 oz
    Water   2 qts

Dissolve & boil one half hour to make it blue add more pruciate potass

Sr Siewises receipt is 1 oz ext logwood 1 drachm bicarbonate potass 3 qts warm water & mix

Elderberry Wine

Pull the berries from the stalks and put them in a tub. Pour boiling water on them, 2 gallons water to 3 gallons berries. Press them down into the liquor and cover closely. Let remain in 24 hours, press the juice from the berries clean as possible and to every gallon of this juice add 3 lbs of sugar, 1 oz of cloves, 1 oz ginger. Boil 20 minutes, skim thoroughly while still hot. Put it in a cask or stone jug or bottles, fill the jug or cask full, add to every gall one spoonful of new yeast and stir it well together with a stick. Fresh berries and picked in a dry day is best

Good Black Ink

Prussiate potash 24 grains
Bicarbonate potash 12 grains
Extract logwood 1 oz
Water 2 pints
Dissolve and boil one half hour. To make it blue, add more prussiate potash.
Dr. Lewis's receipt is 1 oz extract dogwood, 1 drachm bicarbonate potash 3 quarts warm water and mix.

✗ Obviating Syrup

Senna 6 oz extract butternut 8 oz jalap 3 oz
Liquorice root 2 oz mandrake 2 oz ginger root 2 drachms
Cloves 2 drachms Caraway ½ oz Coriander seed
½ oz anice 1½ oz (13 oz of all the above) to be put
in diluted alcohol enough to cover the medicine
add to the above juniper berries 8 oz iris 4 oz
then let stand often stiring 2 weeks tight covered
strain press out all the spirit add boiling brandy
enough to cover the dregs let stand 24 or 36
hours press & boil the liquor down to a qt
or less and add the spirit first made warm
both togather and add good brown sugar
a lb to the qt bring to a boil skim clean
and bottle to be taken sufficient to keep the
bowels in a healthy condition a good medicine

Chill Fever & Ague

Brandy or Alcohol ½ pt ½ pt molasses
½ lb white sugar 1 drachm Quinine 1 oz Rhei
1 oz Senna 1 oz peruvian bark not pulverised
put the Rhei bark senna in water boil to
get the full strength strain press the drugs
let settle pour of the clear part add the quinine
sugar & molasses alcohol or brandy oil wintergreen

Obviating Syrup

Senna 6 oz, extract butternut 3 oz, jalap 3 oz, licorice root 2 oz, ginger root 2 drachms, cloves 2 drachms, mandrake 2 oz, caraway ½ oz, coriander seed ½ oz, anise 1½ oz (13 oz of all the above) to be put in diluted alcohol enough to cover the medicine. Add to the above juniper berries 8 oz, iris 4 oz. Then let stand, often stirring, 2 weeks tight covered. Strain, press out all the spirit, add boiling brandy, enough to cover the dregs. Let stand 24 or 36 hours, press, and boil the liquor down to a gal or less and add the spirit first—made warm both together and add good brown sugar, a lb to the quart—bring to a boil, skim clean and bottle to be taken sufficient to reef? the bowels in a healthy condition—a good medicine.

Chill Fever and Ague

Brandy or alcohol ½ pint, ½ pint molasses, ½ lb white sugar, 1 drachm quinine, 1 oz rhubarb, 1 oz senna, 1 oz Peruvian bark not pulverized. Put the rhubarb, bark, senna in water, boil it to get the full strength. Strain, press the drugs, let settle, pour off the clear part, add the quinine, sugar and molasses, alcohol or brandy, oil wintergreen

122

of Sasafrass mix all well and take a
table Spoonfull according to circumstances.

{Clapps}

Golden seal root	1 oz
Ginsing root	2 "
Queen of the meadow root	3 oz
Sweet flag root	1 "
Shirknard root	4 "
Sarsaparilla root	4 "
Comfrey root	2 "
burdock seed	3 "

20 oz in all put all in one gall of water
keep hot nearly to boiling point 6 hours then
slowly boil down to 1 qt Strain settle add
1 lb crushed sugar disolve by stiring and
add good gin 1 qt — Doce 2 table Spoon
fulls every 3 hours to be continued often
bathe the parts in cold water

× For Mother Neuralga & pain in the head
My bathing drop 5 oz Aqua ammonia 2 druchms chloraphoum
2 druchms Laudanum 2 druchms mix and bathe the painful
parts often & often smell from the bottle as much as can be
easily borne if neuralgia is hard wet a cloth & apply often wet-
ing it and keep it applied for a good length of time

and sassafras. Mix all well and take a tablespoonful according to circumstances.

Clap

Golden Seal root 1 oz
Ginseng root 2 oz
Queen of the Meadow root 3 oz
Sweet Flag root 1 oz
Spikenard root 4 oz
Sarsaparilla root 4 oz
Comfrey root 2 oz
Burdock seed 3 oz

20 oz in all, put all in on gall of water. Keep hot, nearly to the boiling point 6 hours, then slowly boil down to 1 quart. Strain, settle, add 1 lb crushed sugar, dissolve by stirring and add good gin 1 quart. Dose: 2 tablespoonfuls every 3 hours, to be continued often, bathe the parts in cold water.

For Another Neuralgia and Pain in the Head

My bathing drops 1 oz, aqua ammonia 2 drachms, chloroform 2 drachms, laudanum 2 drachms. Mix and bathe the painful parts often and often smell from the bottle as much as can be easily done if neuralgia is hard. Wet a cloth and apply often. Wetting it and keep it applied for a good length of time.

Itch Ointment x

One plug tobacco one handful catnip a spoonful pepper dittio Salt, little ginger 2 tea spoonfulls Sulpher one lb fresh butter or lard with a little mutton tallow boil the catnip and tobacco in splts to git all the strength simmer the lard untill the watter disapears then add the other articles pulverised.

Plaster x

3½ pts. sweet oil or fresh butter when biled and skimed 1 pt linseed oil boil theme in a skillet so hot that it will burn a feather then add 1 lb pulverizied Red lead to be stirred gently in to it while hot but the oil must be a little cooled or it will boil over. Uses Old sores gangrenous ulcers on the legs or elswhere or fresh cuts or wounds are ket-together and united by healing + Fever Sore ♃ Honey and casteel soap equie parts to be applied and occasiunly the follening Bosilicon ℥j Calleemen ℥j mix

Itch Ointment

One plug tobacco, one handful catnip, a spoonful pepper, ditto salt., little ginger, 2 teaspoonfuls sulfur, one lb fresh butter or lard with a little mutton tallow. Boil the catnip and tobacco in spirits to get all the strength, simmer the lard until the water disappears, then add the other articles pulverized.

Plaster

3½ pints sweet oil or fresh butter when boiled and skimmed, 1 pint linseed oil, boil them in a skillet so hot that it will burn a feather. Then add 1 lb pulverized red lead to be stirred gently into it while hot, but the oil must be a little cooled or it will boil over. Uses: old sores, gangrenous ulcers on the legs or elsewhere, or fresh cuts or wounds are ret-together and united by healing.

Fever Sore

Honey and Castile Soap equal parts to be applied and occasionally the following: Bosilicon[245] ℥j [℥=ounce], Calamine ℥j, mix.

---

[245] Ceratum resinae, rosin cerate

✗ Clap or Gonorrhoea

Bathe the parts daily with luke warm water wiping away all the secretions — rest from labor live lower than usual. take once a week a dose of senna manna & salts. Drink daily of toast & water barley water &c & flax seed tea avoid salted or high seasoned meats & all ardent spirits the urine becomes less irritating and the scalding less
℞ ♃ 11 ℈ ♃ ♀ ♄ ct i, ♃ ♃ ℥ Apply a cold poultice of oat meal or slipery elm moistened with vinegar or Gollards extract of lead renewed 3 or 4 times a day take every other day a dose of salts if this does not reduce the swelling apply 6 or 8 leaches if very painful take 20 drops every 2 hours ℞

✗ Gleet ‒ use injections of sugar of lead & white vitrol not strong twice a day a tea spoonful of peruvian bark in Port wine may be taken twice a day Cold bathing with a sponge on the small of the back and about the genitals avoid to early ♃ ♀ ♀ ♃ ♃ ♃ i ℥ ℞ ⟨⟩ ♃ ♀ ♀ ♀ ♃ ♃ inject a little sweet oil or flax

Clap or Gonorrhea

Bathe the parts daily with lukewarm water, wiping away all the secretions—rest—from labor, live lower than usual. Take once a week a dose of senna manna and salts. Drink daily of teas and water, barley water or flaxseed tea. Avoid salted or high seasoned meats and all ardent spirits. The urine becomes less irritating and the scalding less.

Swelled Testicle[246]

Apply a cold poultice of oatmeal or slippery elm, moistened with vinegar or Gollard's extract—of lead renewed 3 or 4 times a day. Take every other day a dose of salts. If this does not reduce the swelling apply 6 or 8 leeches. If very painful take 20 drops every 2 hours.

Gleet

Use injections of sugar lead and white vitriol, not strong, twice a day a teaspoonful of Peruvian bark in Port wine may be taken twice a day. Cold bathing with a sponge on the small of the back and about the genitals. Avoid too early CONNECTION WITH WOMEN inject a little sweet oil or flax

---

246 Translated from code

seed tea milk warm

Phymosis ♂ immerse the g[l]ans several times a day in milk warm water and in sweet oil or a decoction of mallows root & flax seed also inject the same under the freskin or between the preface and glands apply a paultice of milk & bread or slipery elm

Paraphymosis ♂ the same application as to phymosis if these should not suesued apply cloths diped in [symbols] or a [symbols] applied [symbols] take [symbols]

Pain Killer ♂ Alcohol 1 gall Gum Camphor 12 lb oil origanum & oil Hemlock each 8 oz oil turpentine & oil Cayenne each 1 oz oil Sassafras & pepermint & spearmint each 2 oz — mix use externaly and take internaly teaspoonful doses ½ for rheumatism acute & chronic — nervous sprains — stiffness of joints chilblains swellings white swellings pain in joints and sprain of all discriptions & characters

seed tea milk warm.

Phimosis

Immerse the penis[247] several times a day in milk, warm water and in sweet oil or a decoction of mallows root or flaxseed, also inject the same under the foreskin or between the prepuce and glands. Apply a poultice of milk and bread or slippery elm.

Paraphimosis

The same application as to phimosis if those should not succeed. Apply cloths dipped in brandy cold vinegar or a cold poultice applied.[248]

Tight Erections[249]

Take cannab and immerse in cold vinegar in water.[250]

Pain Killer

Alcohol 1 gallon, gum camphor ½ lb, oil origanum and oil hemlock each 8 oz, oil turpentine and oil cayenne each 1 oz, oil sassafras and peppermint and spearmint each 2 oz. Mix. Use externally and take internally teaspoonful doses for rheumatism acute and chronic nervous, sprains, stiffness of joints, chilblains, swellings, white swellings, pain in joints and sprains of all descriptions and characters.

---

247 Translated from code
248 Translated from code
249 Translated from code
250 Translated from code

126

Cholic) White root peppermint smart weed taken freely Bath th feet &c

Stomack Pills 1 oz Extract peach leave one teaspoonful cayenne lobelia seed pulverised ½ oz two teaspoonfuls nerve powder five drops Oil peppermint pennyroyal or spearmint

Annother lobelia seed 4 oz nerve powders Caynne 1 oz soda or saleratus 1 oz casteel soap sufficient quantity mix Dose from one to 3 spoonfulls

Strengthning plaster Melt 2 oz Rosin add tea spoonfull cayenne leave to make it of the right consistance.

Plaster for old sores ½ pt linseed oil the same of sweet oil ½ pd red lead simmer slowly to a plaster not burn

Mothers Relief One berry vine ½ pd each of high cranbery or cramp bark and unicorn root ¼ pd blue cohush 1 lb flax seed and red Rosbery leaves each ½ pd pulverise boil in three gall water reduce to 1 and ½ gall add 4 lbs loof sugar half gall good holand gin, dose. half a wine glass 3 times a day for 2 or 3 weeks before confinement

For the blood. Good Sasphrilia 1 lb Sasaphas bark 1 lb Elder flowers 1 lb bone set 2 oz good wood 4 oz green osier ½ pd Yellow Osier 4 oz make 6 qts add 8 lbs sugar 1 qt pure sptr 1 oz Iodide potassa

Colic

White root, peppermint, smartweed taken freely, Bathe. Dr. feet.

Stomach Pills

1 oz extract peach leave one seed pulverized ½ oz, two teaspoonfuls nerve powder, press drops oil peppermint, pennyroyal, or spearmint.

Another

Lobelia seed 4 oz, nerve powders cayenne 1 oz, soda or saleratus 1 oz, castile soap sufficient quantity, mix. Dose from one to 3 spoonfuls.

Strengthening Plaster

Melt 2 oz Rosin, add teaspoonful cayenne, lard to make it of the right consistency.

Plaster for old sores

½ pint linseed oil, the same of sweet oil, ½ pd red lead. Simmer slowly to a plaster, not burn.

Mother's Relief

One berry vine ½ pd each of high cranberry or cramp bark and unicorn root ¼ pd, blue cohosh 1 lb, flaxseed and red raspberry leaves each ½ pd. Pulverize, boil in three gall water, reduce to 1½ gall, add 4 lbs loaf sugar, half gall good holland gin. Dose: half a wine glass 3 times a day for 2 or 3 weeks before confinement.

For the blood—Good

Sarsaparilla 1 lb, sassafras bark 1 lb, elder flowers 1 lb bone set 2 oz, guaiac wood 4 oz, green oxide ½ pd, yellow rosin 4 oz, make 6 quarts add 2 lbs sugar 1 quart pure spirits, 1 oz Iodide Potash

Catarrh Snuff — Blood root ʒj
mix well made very fine Skunk Cabbage ʒj
add oil bergamont oil Canada snake root or
lavender oil lemon Aarabaxca ʒj
oil rosemary to scent Cayenne pepper 20 grs
with for Catarrh pain Bitter root ʒj
in the head tightness Pulverised Liquorice ʒiij
of the head sore eyes Bayberry ʒj
from obstructions in Turpeth mineral ʒj
the head keep in tight White helebore ʒj
stoped bottles this is a very good medicine

× Lucy's Cold bitters ⅔ American Gencian
Luoscea orange peel & ginger Columbea with a
few drops of essence wintergreen ⅔

Adhesive Plaster ⅔ White rosen 18½ oz 1½ oz mutton
tallow loaf or crushed sugar 1 table spoonfull to be
added when warm   × Currant Wine
13 lbs sugar 16 gals water 8 gallons currant
juice 1½ gal best brandy put the brandy in after
the fermentation or after the fermentation has
gone on two weeks or even 10 days will doo.
For Worms ⅔ burn worm wood not to ashes but to blackness
on a shovel or sheet iron mix in bulk 3 parts of the ashes
and one of the carbonate magnetic. Dose from one half
to a tea spoon full repeat

Catarrh Snuff

Bloodroot ℨj [ℨ=ounce]
Skunk cabbage ℨj
Canada snake root or arabica ℨj
Cayenne pepper 20 grains
Bitterroot ℨj
Pulverized licorice ℨjjj
Bayberry ℨj
Turpeth mineral[251] ℨj
White Hellebore ℨ

Mix well made very fine, add oil bergamot, oil lavender, oil lemon, oil rosemary to scent, with for catarrh pain in the head, tightness of the head, sore eyes from obstructions in the head. Keep in tight stopped bottles. This is very good medicine.

Lucy's Cold Bitters

American Ginseng, Quassia orange peel and ginger Columbia with a few drops of essence wintergreen

Adhesive Plaster

White rosin 13 ½ oz, 1½ oz mutton tallow, loaf or crushed sugar 1 tablespoonful to be added when warm.

Currant Wine

73 lbs sugar, 16 gals water 8 gallons currant juice, 1½ gal best brandy. Put the brandy in after the fermentation or after the fermentation has gone on two weeks or even 10 days will do.

For Worms

Burn worm wood not to ashes but to blackness on a shovel or sheet iron, mix in bulk 3 parts of the ashes and one of the carbonates magnetic. Dose from one half to a teaspoonful. Repeat.

---

251 Mercury oxonium sulfate

128

X For Costive habits
Jalop ℈j soap ℈j puff goll properly done away to the thickness of tar formed in to pills
Comp lineament of Stillingia No 1, oil cajeput – ½ fluid oz oil Lobelia 2 fluid drachms oil Stillingia 1 fluid oz ʒ No 2. Oil Stillingia Rectified oil amber each one fluid oz oil Lobelia 3 fluid oz olive oil 2 fluid oz mix ʒ Properties & uses Chronic Asthma Croup Cholera Epilepsy Rheumatism Sciatica & in Chorea & spasmodic diseases the whole vertebral column is to be bathed with it as well as Rheumatism & painful afflictions &c it is prompt & effectual ʒ No 1 it cures the most obstinate cases of Asthma when used about the face & neck it will be tasted the next day in many cases it may be applied every hour or half hour & continued until vomiting ensues it acts as a stimulant relaxant & antispasmodic often affecting a cure without any internal medicine ʒ for the tuth to be used with the above receipt to clean the tuth after using powdered rhatany root myrrh & cream tarter

& Pill Coating) Take flax seed 1 part Loaf sugar 3 parts Spring Sufficient quantity a thick mucelage is obtained by carefully boiling the seeds the sugar is added and the whole of the moisture is evaporated by careful disication this mixture may be reduced to very fine powder and employed for covering the pills sugar Sugar of milk and starch and a little very fine Gum Arabec may be added if thought proper

For Captive Habits

Jalop? Ɔj [Ɔ=scruple], soap Ɔj, beefs gall properly done away to the thickness of tar form into pills

Comp Liniment of Stillingia

No. 13 oil cajeput ½ fluid oz, oil lobelia 2 fluid drachms, oil Stillingia 1 fluid oz, No 2 oil Stillingia, rectified oil amber, each one fluid oz, oil lobelia 3 fluid oz, olive oil 2 fluid oz. Mix. Properties and uses chronic asthma, dyspepsia, rheumatism, sciatica, Croup, Cholera and in cholera and spasmodic diseases. The whole vertebral column to be bathed with it as well as rheumatism and painful afflictions. It is prompt and effectual. No 1, it cures the most obstinate cases of asthma when used about the face and neck. It will be tasted the next day in many cases. It may be applied every hour or half hour and continued until vomiting ensues. It acts as a stimulating relaxant and antispasmodic often effecting a cure without any internal medicine. For the latter to be used with the above recipe. To clean the teeth after using. Powdered rhoting? root, myrrh, and cream tartar.

Pill Coating

Take flaxseed 1 part, loaf sugar 3 parts, spring sufficient quantity a thick mucilage is obtained by carefully boiling the seeds. The sugar is added and to the whole of the moisture is evaporated by careful desiccation of this mixture, may be reduced to very fine powder, and employed for curing the pills. Sugar, sugar of milk and starch and a little very fine gum Arabic may be added if though prepped.

Index to this Book

Diarrhoea	114
Hydro Alcoholic ext Blue cohush	115
Vegitable drops	116
Comp tinc lobelia	117
Syrup of wild chery	117
Comp Syrup of Rheubarb	118
Indian Lineament	169
Elderbery wine	120
Good black ink	120
Oviating Syrup	121
Chill fever and ague	124
Clapp	122
For Mothers Neuralgea and pain in head	122
Itch ointment	123
Plaster	123
Fever sore	123
Clapp or Gonnorrhoea	124
Swelled testicle	124
Gleet	124
Phymosis	125
Paraphymosis	125

Index to this Book

* Note: Please go by the original numbers at the top of the original page scans

Diarrhea	114
Hydro Alcoholic ext Blue Cohosh	115
Vegetable Drops	116
Comp Tinc Lobelia	117
Syrup of Wild Cherry	117
Comp Syrup of Rhubarb	118
Indian Liniment	119
Elderberry Wine	120
Good Black Ink	120
Obviating Syrup	121
Chill fever and Ague	121
Clap	122
For Mother, Neuralgia, and pain in the head	122
Itch Ointment	123
Plaster	123
Fever Sore	123
Clap or Gonorrhea	124
Swelled Testicle	124
Gleet	124
Phimosis	125
Paraphimosis	125

Night Erection	125
Pain Killer	125
Cholic	126
Stomach pills	126
Annotto	126
Strengthing plastr	126
plastr for old sores	126
Mothers relief	126
for the flood	126
Catarrh Snuff	127
Lucys cold Bitters	127
Currant Wine	127
for worms	127
Costive habits	128
No 1	128
No 2	128
Properties & uses	128
For Ringworm my best linneament	47
Cancer plastr	48
Pain in Stomah Bowels	48
Diptheria	48
Rheumatic Linneament	48
pill coatings	128

Night Erection	125
Pain Killer	125
Colic	126
Stomach Pills	126
Another	126
Strengthening Plaster	126
Plaster for old sores	126
Mother's relief	126
For the blood	126
Catarrh snuff	127
Lucy's cold bitters	127
Currant Wine	127
For worms	127
For Costive Habits	128
No. 1	128
No. 2	128
Properties and uses	128
For ringworm	47
My best liniment	47
Cancer plaster	48
Pain in stomach bowels	48
Diphtheria	49
Rheumatic liniment	49
Pill coating	128

Index tt this book

Adhesive Plaster	41
Cough med	41
Eye Water	42
For the Croup	42
Staining Guns	42
For the Croup by B F Hall	43
For the Dropsy by "	43
Green Salve by B F Hall	43
Stomach Bitters by "	44
Bathing Drops " "	44
Phisodgin for coughs &c	45
Laceys Ague Bitters	45
To remove Pimples from face	45
Dr Hals best liniment	46
Eye Water	46
~~Good Bier~~	47
Tooth Ache	50
Itch ointment	50
Fit drops	50
Healing Salve	51
Worms	51
Blue Cohosh and its properties	51

Adhesive plaster	41
Cough medicine	41
Eye Matter	42
For the Croup	42
Staining Guns	42
For the Croup by B. F. Hale	43
For the Dropsy by B. F. Hale	43
Green Salve by B. F. Hale	43
Stomach Bitters by B. F. Hale	44
Bathing Drops by B. F. Hale	44
Phloridzin for Coughs	45
Lucy's Ague Bitters	45
To remove pimples from the face	45
Dr. Hale's best liniment	46
Eye Water	46
~~Good Beer~~	47
Toothache	50
Itch Ointment	50
Fit Drops	50
Healing Salve	51
Worms	51
Blue Cohosh and its properties	51

Luceys Ague Bitters	51
Cough Balsam	51
Nerve and Bone Lineament	52
Cough Powders	52
Worm Lozenges	53
Rheumatic Lineament	54
For the lungs and cough	54
Cholera Med	55
Grand Ague Med	55
Cornes	55
Black Salve	56
Cologn water	57
Green Salve	57
Sweet Tinct Rheubarb	57
Luceys last cough med	57
Hydrophobia	58
Diarrhoea	58
Anrothu	58
Alterative	59
Stomach Bitters or Cordial	59
D Halls Samaritan Lineament	60
Mothers very excelent med for pain in Stomach bowels	61
Discutient Ointment	61

Lucy's Ague Bitters	51
Cough Balsam	51
Nerve and bone liniment	52
Cough powders	52
Worm Lozenges	53
Rheumatic liniment	54
For the lungs and cough	54
Cholera Med	55
Grand Ague Med	55
Corns	55
Black Salve	56
Cologne Matter	57
Gran Salve	57
Sweet Tinct Rhubarb	57
Lucy's last cough med	57
Hydrophobia	58
Diarrhea	58
Another	58
Alterative	59
Stomach bitters or cordial	59
Dr. Hale's Samaritan liniment	60
Mother's very excellent med for pain in stomach, bowels	61
Discutient Ointment	61

Spasmodic Attack   62

Syrup for lungs   62
Dysmenorrhoe,   63
Cast-liver pill   64
Cough med   64
Dysentric med, Cordial,   65
Dry Cast Ague pills   65
White liquied physic   66
Powerful Nervine   66
Gonorrhoer Injection   66
Another   66, 67
    Gonorrhoea   67
Stomach cordial or bitters   68
Eruption on the face   68
Liver powders   69
Liver drops   69
Simple Cerate   70
Rheumatic Linct   70
The batheing drops   70
Rheumatism   71
Lineament for Sprains &   71
Vermafuge   71

Spasmodic attacks	62
Syrup for lungs	62
Dysmenorrhea	63
Last liver pills	64
Cough med	64
Dysentery med cordial	65
My last Ague pills	65
White liquid physic	66
Powerful nervine	66
Gonorrhea injection	66
Another	66, 67
Gonorrhea	67
Stomach cordial or bitters	68
Eruption on the face	68
Liver powders	69
Liver drops	69
Simple Cerate	70
Rheumatic tinct	70
The bathing drops	70
Rheumatism	71
Liniment for sprains	71
Vermifuge	71

Gonorrhoea	72
For tape worm	73
Cologn water	73
Infants Cordial	73
Worms a good vermifuge	74
Cough med	74
Lip Salve	75
For Cough	75
Eye wash	75
To remove flims	75
Sticking Salve	75
Dr Hales Cholera Syrup	76
Black Linneament	76
Pomade for restoreing the hair	77
Vervine and carminative balsam	77
Conklins Salve	78
Lords Salve	78
Cholera drops	78
For injection in Leucorrhoer Gonnorh	78
Pain killer	79
For goiter Swelled neck Scrofulous cancers	79
Eye Watter. Grandfathers best.	80
Dirheoa and Cholera Mortus	80

Gonorrhea	72
For tape worm	73
Cologne matter	73
Infant's cordial	73
Worms, a good vermifuge	74
Cough med	74
Lip salve	75
For cough	75
Eye Wash	75
To remove films	75
Sticking salve	75
Dr. Hale's Cholera syrup	76
Black liniment	76
Pomade for restoring the hair	77
Nervine and carminative balsam	77
Conklin's salve	78
Lord's salve	78
Cholera drops	78
For injection in leukorrhea, gonorrhea	78
Pain killer	79
For goiter, swelled neck, scrofulous cancers	79
Eye water, grandfather best	80
Diarrhea and cholera morbus	80

	135
Salt Rheum Ointment	81
Pills for Dropsy	81
Emmenagogue tinct	81
Spice Bitters	82
Cytaneous cancers	82
Comp tinct Camphor	82
Pery davises pain killer	83
Wtridge nerve ointment	83
Bone Linneament	83
Scrofula pill	84
comp tinct camphor Rheumatic drops or Painkiller	84
Chilblains	85
Dr Allens cholera Syrup	85
Comp Ointment Stramonium	86
Comp wine of Comfry	86
For cough	87
Nerve and bone linneament	87
Dyspeptic Powders	88
Cutaneous Ointment	88
Cough Balsam	88
Lavender Watter	89
Hungary Water	89

Salt rheum ointment	81
Pills for Dropsy	81
Emmenagogue tinct	81
Spice Bitters	82
Cutaneous cancers	82
Comp tinct camphor	82
Pery Davis's pain killer	83
Kitridge nerve ointment	83
Bone liniment	83
Scrofula pill	84
Comp tinct camphor, rheumatic drops, or pain killer	84
Chilblains	85
Dr. Allen's cholera syrup	85
Comp ointment stramonium	86
Comp wine of Comfrey	86
For cough	87
Nerve and bone liniment	87
Dyspeptic powders	88
Cutaneous ointment	88
Cough balsam	88
Lavender water	89
Pulmonary water	89

Index

	page
Canker	1
Vegetable powder	1
Wallis Cough med	2
No 6	3
Vegetable Bitters	3
do Ointment	4
do Syrup for Disentary	4
Worm Syrup	5
Disentary	5
Cough Emulsion	6
Sore Eyes	6
Lees Pill	7
Quick pill No 1	7
Ague Pill	7
Ague Pill	7
For Corns	8
Palmonary Mixture	8
Venerial ɔɔ x q	9
Spruice Beer	9
Diarhoea	10
Hiera Picra	10
Cough drops	10

Index

Vegetable physic	10
Spruice Beer	11
Itch Ointment	11
Compound Balsom	11
g o t Medicine	12
Cure for Gravel	12
Good for the Itch	12
Ague Bitters	12
For Bots & Belly Ache	13
Itch Ointment	13
Medical or Root Beer	13
Rhumatic Liniment	14
Black Salve	14
Best Adhesive Plaster	15
Fever & Ague	15
Ammenagogue	16
For Gonnorrhoea or Clap	16
My Emetic	17
Burnes, Scalds, cuts wounds of any kinds	18
Diarrhoea	18
Purgantia Pill	19

Index

Canker	1
Vegetable powder	1
Wallis Cough Med	2
No. 5	3
Vegetable Bitters	3
do ointment	4
do Syrup for Dysentery	4
Worm Syrup	5
Cough Emulsion	6
Sore Eyes	6
Lee's Pill	7
Quick Pill No. 1	7
Ague Pill	7
Ague Pill	7
For Corns	8
Pulmonary Mixture	8
Venereal CLAP	9
Spruce Beer	9
Hiera Picra	10
Cough Drops	10

Index

Vegetable Physic	10
Spruce beer	11
Itch Ointment	11
Compound Balsam	11
g o x Medicine	12
Cure for gravel	12
Good for the itch	12
For bots and belly ache	13
Itch ointment	13
Medical or Root Beer	13
Rheumatic liniment	14
Black Salve	14
Best adhesive plaster	15
Fever and ague	15
Emmenagogue	16
For Gonorrhea or Clap	16
My Emetic	17
Burns, scalds, cuts, wounds of any kind	18
Diarrhea	18
Purgantia Pill	19

Palpitation	89
Bitters	90
Ointment for the eye	90
Cough Drops	90
Annother and a better	91
Cough powders	91
For Cholera and Cholera morbus	92
Plaster sticking	92
Linniament for people	92
" " horses	92
Sure cure for Hydrophobia	93
Cornes	93
For piles	93
Hellenium Balsam	94
For Neuralgia	94
Cholera med	95
Kitriges Nerve Ointment	95
To prepare soap	95
Female weakness	95
Salve	96
Rheumatism tried	96
Kitriges Ointment	97
For Dysentary or diarrhoea	97

Palpitation	89
Bitters	90
Ointment for the eye	90
Cough Drops	90
Another and a better	91
Cough powders	91
For Cholera and Cholera morbus	92
Plaster sticking	92
Liniment for people or horses	92
Sure cure for hydrophobia	93
Corns	93
For piles	93
Helenium Balsam	94
For Neuralgia	94
Cholera med	95
Kitridges Nerve Ointment	95
To prepare soap	95
Female weakness	95
Salve	96
Rheumatism tinct	96
Kitridges Ointment	97
For dysentery or diarrhea	97

138
3

Cement for cisterns	98	Horse and man lineaments	105
Godfreys cordial	98		
Wallaces Cough Med	98	Dyptheria	105
Quinzy	98	Cost Alterative	106
Cologn	99	Hair dye	106
Affections of the Spleen	99	A nnother	106
Remidy called Cureall	99	Stregnting plaster	106
and part of this is on the	100	Cost Alterative	107
Bleeding of the Lungs	67	Chronic Rheumatism	108
Fever Sores	67	Sudorific drops that	
Rheumatic Lineament	49	belong to the Chronic	
Oint for tinea capitis	100	Rheumatism Recpt and	
Blister plaster	100	to no other	108
Linneament Sacred	100	Sudorific drops	108
Stramonium Oint	101	Infection for Gohnorhoea	109
Staining gun Barrels	131	Vegtable Salve	109
to case harden	102	Fever Lungs & blood	109
Emmory	102	Lineament for Scofula	110
Cooling plaster	102	Chery pectoral	110
Indian Salve	102	R for making vegitabl. Oil	111
for Ague and fever	103	Comp Saksapilleiu	111
Composition Improved	103	to Mertia colivation	112
Alterative	103	Gonnorhoea	112
liver Syrup	104	Lungs & liver	113

Cement for cisterns	98	Horse and man liniment	105
Godrey's cordial	98		
Wallace Cough med	98	Diphtheria	105
Quinsy	99	Last alterative	106
Cologne	99	Hair dye	106
Afflictions of the spleen	99	Another	106
Remedy called cure all	99	Strengthening Plaster	106
and part of this is in the	100	last alterative	107
Bleeding of the lungs	67	Chromic Rheumatism	108
Fever sores	67	Sudorific drops that belong to the chronic rheumatism recpt and to no other	108
Rheumatic liniment	49		
Oint for tinea captis	100		
Blister plaster	100		
Liniment sacred	100	Sudorific drops	108
Stramonium ointment	101	Infection for gonorrhea	109
Staining gun barrels	101	Vegetable salve	109
To case harden	102	Liver Lungs and blood	109
Emory	102	Liniment for scrofula	110
Cooling plaster	102	Cherry pectoral	110
Indian Salve	102	Rx for making veg oil	111
For ague and fever	103	Comp sarsaparilla	111
Composition improved	103	to produce salivation	112
Alterative	103	Gonorrhea	112
Liver syrup	104	Limes liver	118

No 2

	Page		Page
Cookies	21	Harrison cake	26
Another	21	Cream cake	27
Wafers	21	Sunderland pudding	27
Jumbles	21	Pound Cake	27
Cookies	22	Kings cake	27
Nut cake	22	Indelible Ink	27
Muffins	22	To colour Green	28
Number Cake	22	Pound cake	28
Rusk	22	Pudding	28
Measure Cake	23	Birds nest pudding	29
Little Cake	23	Gingerbread	29
Sponge Cake	23	Cider cake	29
Plumb Cake	23	Bread	30
Crackers	24	To Cure warts	30
Ginger Bread	24	Soft Gingerbread	30
Fruit cake	24	Cookies	30
Puff paste	24	French Loaf	30
York Biskett	24	Oisters Imitation	31
Whip Syllybub	25	To Clean Gloves	31
Loaf Cake	25	Good Custard	31
Icing for cake	25	To Clean Bed Ticks	32
John bull pudding	26		
Cookies	26		

Cookies	21	Harrison cake	26
another	21	Cream cake	27
Wafers	21	Sunderland pudding	27
Jumbles	21	Pound cake	27
Cookies	22	Kings Cake	27
Nut cake	22	Indelible ink	27
Muffins	22	To color green	28
Number cake	22	Pudding	28
Measure cake	23	Birds Nest Pudding	29
Little cake	23	Gingerbread	29
Sponge cake	23	Cider cake	29
Plums cake	23	Bread	30
Crockers	24	To cure warts	30
Ginger bread	24	Soft Gingerbread	30
Fruit cake	24	Cookies	30
Puff paste	24	French loaf	30
York biscuit	24	Oyster imitations	31
Whip syllabub	25	To clean gloves	31
Loaf cake	25	Good custard	31
Icing for cake	25	To clean bed ticks	32
John Bull pudding	26		
Cookies	26		

```
 5000 Rats   — 25    125000
 1500 Minks  475    7125 0
  900 Coon  100
  150 Pan   600     900 00
 1500 Deer  123     750 00
 1500 Bear 2500    2250
                   32500
 1500
  425             28500
  7500
 10500
  6000
 71,2500

         1150    3)28350(94,346
         7500        27
                     13
 1500               12
  125   1500        15
 7500   2500        15
  500    750000     5
 22500   3000       5
        32,50000    20
                    88
                    2
```

W. S. Hale's Book

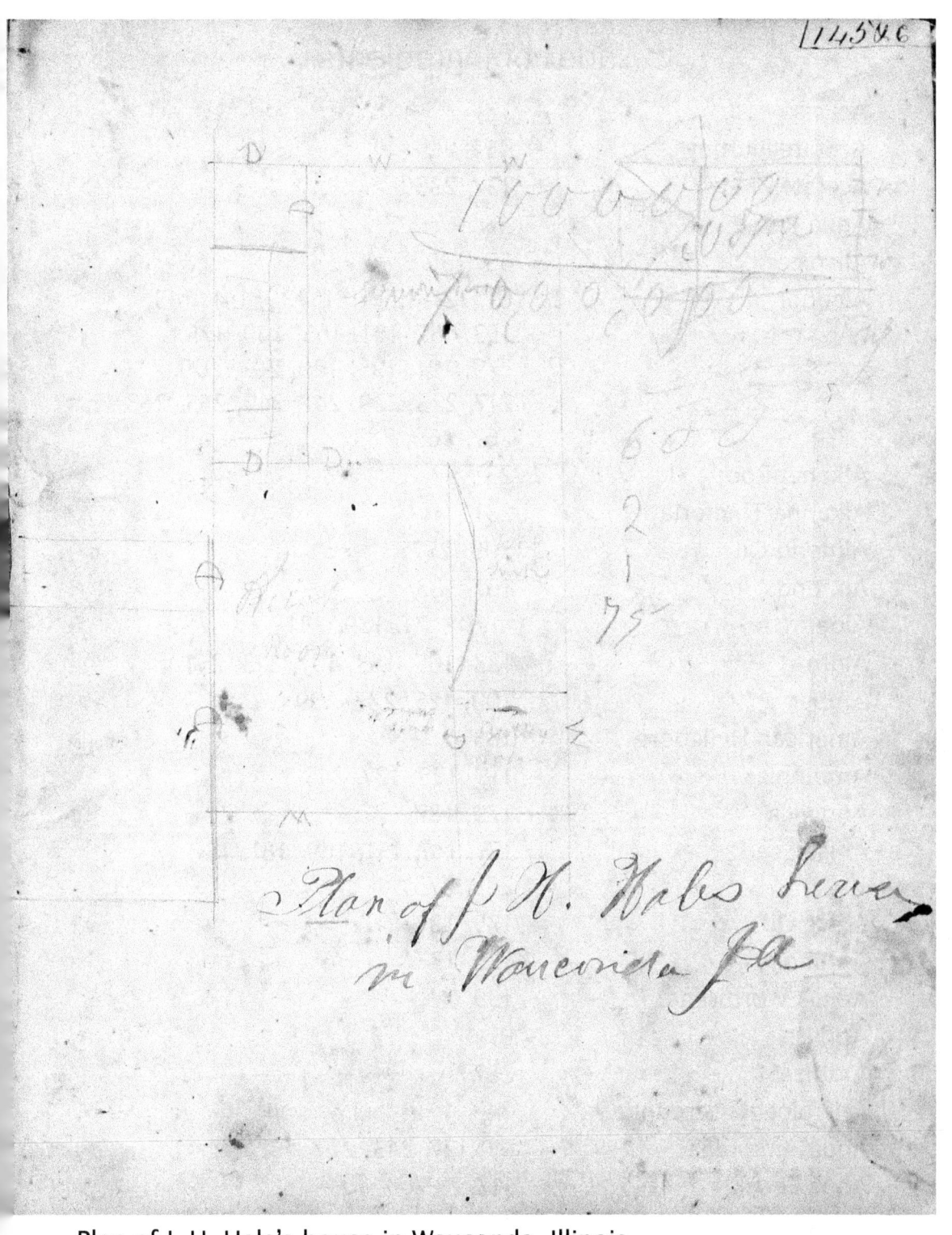

Plan of J. H. Hale's house in Wauconda, Illinois.

Index of Ingredients

Acacia	121
Acetate Plumby	45
Acetate Zinc	127, 233
Agua Purae	45
Allspice	55, 195
Alcohol	61, 121–127, 131, 135, 141, 145, 153, 157, 161, 165, 169, 175, 179, 191, 195, 199, 201, 209, 217, 223–229, 247, 249, 255, 263, 267, 269, 283
Alkanet Root	231
Alkanna Tinctoria	231
Almond Oil	209, 257
Almonds	167, 183
Aloes	41, 47, 71, 179, 231
Alum	123, 165, 183, 197, 243, 251
Amber	109, 125, 227, 289
American Hellebore	165
Ammonia	115, 125, 127, 245
Angelica	179, 187
Anise Seed	121, 147, 151, 169, 181, 187, 259, 275
Anise Oil	175, 181, 217
Antimony	123, 137
Apella Wormseed	139
Apples	91
Arabica	287
Aristolochia serpentiaria	249
Aqua Ammoniac	93, 127, 243, 277
Aqua Fortis	117, 235
Arsenic	47

Asafetida	41, 179
Asarum Canadense	267
Astragalus	197
Baneberry	65
Balm Gilead	225
Balmony	179
Balsam	51–55, 65, 135, 167, 177, 209, 215, 247, 257
Barley Water	281
Bathing Drops	127
Bay Rum	247
Bayberry	35, 39, 41, 143, 227, 239, 287
Beech's Pulmonary Balsam	215
Beef Gall	61, 131, 141, 179, 199, 289
Beef Suet	85, 89
Beer	69
Beeswax	63, 69, 119, 133, 147, 183, 189, 217, 225, 227, 233, 235, 245
Beich Dysenteric Cordial	217
Belladonna	271
Benzian Flowers	207
Benzoic Acid	211
Bergamot	145, 179, 183, 187, 209, 231, 287
Beth Root	223
Bicarbonate Potash	163, 273
Bitter Herb	179
Bitterroot	135, 259, 287
Bitters	135
Bittersweet	41, 57, 155, 199, 205, 241, 247, 255
Bitterwood	213
Black Alder	59
Black Bugbane	65

Black Hellebore	195
Black Pepper	63, 143, 195, 197, 233, 243
Black Snakeroot	65
Blackberry Root	163, 227, 261
Blackroot	57, 171, 251
Block Tin	237
Bloodroot	37, 47, 51, 57, 119, 123, 135, 137, 141, 147, 157, 161, 173, 175, 181, 207, 213, 215, 219, 221, 229, 241, 251, 253, 259, 263, 287
Blue Flag	151, 171, 179, 241, 251, 255–259
Blue Mass	231
Blue Vitriol	117, 193, 235
Bole Armanium	217
Boneset	143, 285
Borage	231
Borax	123, 195, 223, 267
Bosilicon	279
Boxwood	143
Brandy	41, 53, 57, 115, 135, 143, 173, 189, 193, 197, 217, 223, 223, 227, 239, 261, 263, 269, 275, 287
Bread	283
British Oil	55
Buge Weed	259
Burdock	49, 59, 65, 177, 239, 277
Burgundy Pitch	59, 63, 245
Burnt Sponge	201
Butter	133, 147, 219, 279
Butter Resin	59
Butternut	275
Cajeput Oil	141, 197, 201, 217, 289

Calamine	213
Calamus	179, 187
Calcined Copperas	167
Calcium Hydroxide	139
Calomel	47, 233
Camphine Oil	99, 105
Camphor (Gum or Spirits)	61, 125, 127, 133, 137, 141, 143, 149 153, 167, 175, 177, 183, 187–193, 199, 203, 207, 217, 231, 235, 237, 253, 257, 271, 283
Canada Balsam	177
Canada Snake Root	143
Canella	53
Cannabis	165, 283
Cantharides	61, 93, 137, 141, 187, 195, 207, 253
Capsicum	61, 67, 141, 149, 153, 157, 161, 175, 181, 203
Caraway Seed	73, 91, 187, 241, 275
Carbonate of Ammonia	127
Carbonate of Iron	221
Carbonate Magnetic	287
Carbonate Potash	139, 151, 185, 195, 203, 229, 269
Carbonate Soda	177
Cardamom	151, 187
Carnation	231
Carrots	69
Caryophyllum	231
Castile Soap	61, 141, 279, 285
Castor Oil	175, 181, 183
Catechu	121
Catnip	133, 163, 179, 187, 225, 279
Caustic Potash	267

Cayenne	35, 37, 39, 47, 67, 121, 127, 131, 137, 141, 149, 155, 161, 163, 185, 189–201, 209, 215, 217, 223, 235, 239, 271, 283–287
Cedar	111, 125
Chalk	111
Chamomile	41, 67, 205
Chateaux	41, 179
Chelone Glabra	227
Chamber Lye	59, 123, 141, 151, 165, 181, 221
Cherry Bark	241 253, 259, 267
Cherry Wine	157
Chimaphila	65
China Bark	121
Chinchona bark	121
Chloroform	121, 127, 153, 277
Cholic Root	239
Cicuta Leaves	155, 199, 205
Cinnamon	77, 95, 121, 145, 151, 163, 169, 179, 197, 213, 227, 231, 261, 269
Citric Acid	197
Cloves	35, 111, 145, 157, 179, 211, 213, 217, 239, 273, 275
Clove Pink	231
Cocash	175, 259
Cochineal	179
Cognac Brandy	39
Cohosh	65, 67, 123, 135, 141, 173, 175, 181, 195, 225, 239, 249, 259, 263, 285
Colchicum Seed	225
Colocynth	47, 71
Cologne Water	99

Collyrium	193
Colombo	205
Comfrey	37, 137, 147, 161, 205, 215, 221–225, 229, 259, 277
Composition	57, 135, 239, 263
Conium Maculatum	211
Copaiba	65, 167, 177
Copper Carbonate	119
Copper Filings	149
Copper Sulfate	117
Copperas	169
Coriander Seed	121, 213, 275
Corn Meal	73, 95
Corrosive Sublimate	117, 127, 129, 235
Cramp Bark	157, 179, 285
Cranberry	285
Cranesbill	163
Cream Tartar	53, 93, 95, 219
Crocus Martis	125, 167
Croton Oil	161, 175, 181, 195, 197
Culver's Root	53, 171, 251, 259
Curcuma	255
Currants	79, 81, 85, 89, 287
Custard	91
Cyanide	133
Dandelion	63
Devil's Snare	155
Diacylum	63
Digitalis	37, 141, 181, 213, 215, 221, 229, 259
Dogwood	97, 273
Egg	129
Egg Shells	57

Elder Flowers	151, 183, 241, 247, 255, 259, 285
Elder Green	225
Elder Bark	81, 109
Elder Roots	195, 251
Elderberry Wine	273
Elecampane	137, 157, 161, 215, 221, 229, 241, 251, 259
Emetic tart	71
Emorine	237
Ergot	65, 195
Ethyl Nitrite	65, 117
Eupatorium perfolatum	143
Fairy Candle	65
Fals Toung	149
Ferrous Sulfate	167, 169
Fir Balsam	135, 177, 209, 247, 257
Fire Weed	167, 219
Flaxseed	49, 53, 57, 281, 285, 289
Flies, Cantharides	61, 93, 137, 141, 187, 195, 207, 233, 253
Foreign Valerian	141
Foxglove	215
Gall	111
Gamboge	47, 71, 161, 195
Garget Root	151, 199, 245–251
Garlic	179
Gelsemium	165
Gentian Root	121, 151, 169, 197, 205
Geranium	163, 227, 261
Gin	181, 221, 241, 249, 277, 285

Ginger	35, 51, 55, 67, 69, 91, 93, 131, 133, 143, 171, 181, 193–197, 227, 267, 273, 275, 279, 287
Gingko	169
Gingseng Root	277, 287
Glucoside	161
Glycoside of Phloretin	123
Golden Seal	57, 135, 165, 209, 243, 259, 263, 269, 277
Gollard's Extract	281
Gouch	121, 127
Green Oxide	285
Guaiac (Goac)	65, 151, 153, 199, 225, 239, 241, 245–251, 255, 285
Gum Ammoniac	219
Gum Arabic	45, 83, 97, 115, 139, 189, 207, 257, 289
Gum Camp	151
Gum Kino	121, 153, 163, 177
Gum Shellac	101
Gutta	189, 211, 231
Hartshorn	105, 131
Helenium Balsam	215, 221
Hellebore	47, 67, 165, 173, 195, 225, 249, 271, 287
Hemlock	35, 121, 125, 127, 153, 155, 191, 197, 201, 211, 217, 227, 271, 283
High Cranberry	157
Hoffman's Anodyne	193
Honey	37, 53, 55, 109, 119, 131, 135, 147, 159, 183, 209, 211, 213, 229, 279
Hops	179

Horehound	37, 51, 143, 221, 229, 259
Hornet's Nest	117
Hydrate Potash	257
Hydriodate Potash	191
Hydrochloric Acid	219
Hydrocyanic Acid	233
Hyoscyamus	159
Ice Cream	71
Indigo	89, 259
Ipecac	49, 123, 159, 163, 211, 215, 231, 253
Iodide Potash	285
Iodine	191, 193, 201
Iris	275
Iris Versicolor	53, 171, 247
Iron Chloride	177
Ivory Black	101
Jalap	195, 275
Jamaican Ginger	143
Jamaican Rum	245
Jawbone of a Dog	149
Jessamine	165
Jesuit's Bark	121
Jimson Weed	155
Julep	289
Juniper Berries	275
Juniperus Sabina	195
Kitridge's Ointment	227
Lady's Slipper	137, 161, 165, 187, 215
Lard	63, 69, 119, 127, 133, 173, 187, 195, 199, 205, 213, 219, 227, 233, 251, 279, 285

Laudanum	121, 123, 127, 131, 141, 143, 149, 155, 161, 175, 181, 189–193, 199, 225, 229, 235, 257, 271, 277
Lavender	131, 145, 155, 179, 211, 249, 287
Lavendulan	231
Laxative	117
Lead	237, 281
Leeches	281
Lemon	49, 69, 71, 95, 103, 139, 145, 179, 183, 231, 287
Leptandrin	64, 69
Licorice	37, 49, 53, 115, 123, 141, 147, 181, 221, 229, 241, 259, 275, 287
Linseed Oil	107, 111, 113, 125, 145, 231, 237, 279, 305
Liniment	121, 125, 141
Litharge (Lead monoxide)	63
Lobelia	37, 49, 51, 67, 119, 123, 137, 159, 161, 183, 185, 203, 207, 209, 213, 215, 229, 235, 245, 285, 289
Logwood	115, 273
Lupulin	63
Mace	87, 89
Macerotin	159
Marshmallow	177
May Apple	119
Malaga Wine	207
Mallows Root	283
Mandrake	47, 53, 67, 119, 151, 157, 171, 179, 195, 251, 257, 259, 275
Mead	103
Melaleuca Leucadendron	141
Mercuric Chloride	117, 127, 129

Mercury Oxonium Sulfate	287
Milk	283, 289
Milkweed	143
Molasses	41, 51, 55, 17, 103, 111, 189, 229, 241, 275
Morphine	159, 165, 207, 253
Moschus	231
Mountain Liver Wort	241
Mucilage	207, 289
Muriate of Iron	177
Muriatic Acid	165
Musk	145, 179, 211
Muscovado Sugar	71, 221
Mustard Seed	233
Mutton Tallow	115, 133, 183, 189, 217, 225, 233, 279, 287
Myrrh	39, 41, 121, 127, 133, 153, 185, 199, 201, 203, 223, 227, 235, 239, 289
Nature Wine	157
Neat's Foot Oil	41, 199, 223
Neroli	145
Nerve Root	235
Nerve Powder	285
Nightshade	155, 199, 205
Nitrate Potash	243
Nitrate Silver	245
Nitre	65, 125, 161
Nitric Acid	117, 139, 165, 235
Nutmeg	211, 223, 227, 261
Nux Vomica	59, 221, 271
Oatmeal	281
Oil Orange	145

Oil Spice	109
Oil Vitriol	243
Olive Oil	55, 133, 137, 145, 183, 185, 207, 209, 217, 253, 289
Onion Seed	141
Onions	179
Opium	45, 47, 121, 125, 127, 137, 185, 203, 215, 221, 231, 249
Orange Peel	87, 121, 151, 169, 197, 213, 287
Origanum	61, 77, 125, 127, 137, 141, 153, 175, 191, 197–201, 207, 217, 233, 253, 271, 283
Otto Rose	211
Oxalic Acid	197, 237
Oxblood Lilies	171
Palo Santo Tree	65
Paraffin	127
Paregoric	53, 115, 149, 163, 187, 213, 215, 229, 261
Peach, Meat, Pits, Leaves	227, 239, 259, 285
Pearlash	73, 81, 87, 89, 91, 93
Peruvian Bark	121, 151, 169, 281
Pennyroyal	209, 285
Peony	187
Pepper	133, 279
Peppermint	47, 53, 143, 149, 163, 185, 191, 193, 203, 217, 223, 227, 269, 271, 283, 285
Piperine	63
Pipsissewa	65, 239, 253, 255
Pitch	111, 133
Phlorizin	123
Plantain	225

Pleurisy Root	179, 239, 267
Podophyllin	119, 161, 195
Poke Berries	173, 175
Poke Root	245–251
Pokeweed Root	151
Poland Starch	97
Pollen of Hops	63
Pond Lilies	35, 223
Poplar	39, 41, 157, 209
Port Wine	281
Potash	173, 191, 193
Potassium Ferrocyanide	237
Potassium Sodium Tartrate	129
Potassium Tartrate	123
Prickly Ash	57, 173, 175, 179, 189, 225, 249, 253, 257
Prucean	163
Prussic Acid	233
Prussiate Of Potash	237, 273
Quassia	213, 287
Queen of the Meadow	195, 277
Quinine	47, 63, 159, 163, 275
Raisins	37, 85, 87, 89, 95, 229
Rectified Spirits Wine	183, 187, 211
Red Cedar	271
Red Lead	145, 237, 279, 285
Red Saunders	115, 123, 127, 153, 197, 213
Red Raspberry Leaves	35, 285
Red Pepper	63
Red Precipitate	59
Raspberry	35
Rhodphialia	171

Rhubarb	53, 69, 111, 147–151, 185, 261, 269, 275
Rochelle Salts	129
Rosa Flora	251
Rose Water	83, 91, 113, 179, 183, 189, 245
Rosemary	137, 145, 179, 207, 211, 231, 253, 255, 287
Rosin	59, 115, 119, 133, 147, 183, 189, 217, 225, 227, 231, 233, 237, 245, 251, 285, 287
Rue	179, 203
Rum	187, 197, 221, 245, 249
Rye Whiskey	173
Saffron	249
Sage	131, 143
Sal ammoniac	45
Salep	47, 53
Saleratus	49, 53, 67, 73, 89, 149, 177, 261, 285
Salt	41, 59, 131, 133, 183, 223, 231, 243, 251, 279, 281
Salt Fish	179
Saltpeter	111, 143, 183, 243
Sanguinarine	171
Sarsaparilla	57, 67, 239, 241, 247, 251–255, 277, 285
Sassafras	59, 61, 65, 67, 103, 121, 127, 131, 141–145, 151, 153, 179, 191, 197, 201, 229, 235, 239, 241, 245, 247, 251, 255, 259, 271, 277, 283, 285
Savin	195
Secale Cornutum	65

Senna	247, 275, 281
Scammony	47, 161, 171
Sherry	205
Silver Nitrate	245
Simple Cerate	127, 129, 173
Simple Syrup	185, 203
Skull Cap	157, 165, 179, 187, 259
Skunk Cabbage	51, 137, 147, 157, 161, 179, 181, 187, 213, 215, 259, 267, 287
Slaked Lime	139
Slippery Elm	49, 57, 157, 253, 267, 281, 283 195, 259, 285
Smart Weed	179
Snake-head	215, 249, 259, 287
Snake Root	195, 223, 231, 237, 289
Soap	69, 103, 105, 285
Soda	205, 223
Solomon Seal	125
Spanish Red Iron Oxide	191, 271, 283, 285
Spearmint	247
Sperit Run	45, 183, 209, 233
Spermaceti	37, 125, 147, 157, 161, 205
Spikenard	213, 215, 221, 229, 241, 259, 277
Spicea	213, 249
Spirit of Ether	193
Spirits	213, 225, 241, 245, 263
Spirits Niter	117, 165, 177, 221, 235, 257
Spruce	51, 55
Squills	221, 259
Stillingia Root	253, 289
Stinking Hellebore	45

Stoidis Foetidus	45
Strangert Spirits	137
Stramonium	155, 159, 163, 165, 199, 205, 219, 235
Strawberry Leaves	163
Strychnine	221
Starch	289
Sudorific Drops	143
Sugar	37, 45, 49, 53, 69, 101, 105, 113, 123, 137, 139–143, 147, 151, 153, 159–163, 169, 171, 181, 183, 187, 193, 197, 209, 227–231 237, 245–249, 253, 257, 261, 267, 269, 273–277, 285–289
Sugar Lead (Lead Acetate)	45, 63, 113, 189, 243, 245, 251 281
Sulfate Morphea	165, 201, 221
Sulfate Soda	165
Sulfate of Magnesia	165
Sulfur	129, 133, 195, 219, 223, 245, 279
Sulfur Lime	189
Sulfur Zinc	63, 113, 125, 167
Sulfuric Acid	55, 115, 185
Sulfuric Ether	131, 155
Swamp Hellebore	271
Sweet Clover	225
Sweet Flag	277
Sweet Oil	53, 237, 243, 255, 257, 265, 281–285
Syrup of Wild Cherry	213, 215
Tag Alder	253
Tamarack Bark	157, 161, 259

Tanner's Oil	243
Tannic Acid	165
Tansy	175, 181
Taraxacum	63
Tar	143, 195
Tartar	67, 69, 151, 195, 289
Tartaric Acid	101, 103, 115
Tetrahydrozoline	193
Thornapple	155
Thoroughwort	39, 67
Thymus Capitatus	121
Tincture of Steel (Iron Chloride)	117, 235
Toad	225
Tobacco	109, 133, 155, 195, 199, 227, 279
Tolu	55, 207
Tragacanth	195
Trillium Erectum	223
Turnip	45, 137, 161, 173, 215
Turpentine	41, 53, 55, 59, 61, 101, 105, 107, 113, 119, 121, 125, 127, 133, 137, 141, 153, 167, 175, 177, 181, 185, 189, 191, 195, 199, 201, 205, 217, 223–227, 231, 243, 253, 255, 271, 283
Turpeth Mineral	287
Unicorn Root	285
Urine	109, 131, 227
Valerian	141, 161, 165, 179, 181, 259
Vanilla	71
Venice Turpentine	205, 227
Vinegar	41, 117, 131, 219, 237, 243, 267, 281
Verdigris	119, 147, 149, 189, 219, 233

Vuburnum opulus	157
Vitriol	45, 61, 63, 89, 107, 117, 129, 141, 213, 243
Wandering Milkweed	143
Wahoo	143, 157, 173
Water Hemlock	155
Wax	173, 237
Whiskey	37, 117, 173, 247
White Hellebore	47, 67, 173, 225, 249, 287
White Oak Bark	163
White Pine Bark	161
White Root	157, 221, 259, 285
White Vitriol (Zinc sulfate)	147, 129, 167, 213, 251, 281
White Wax	173, 183
Wild Cherry Syrup	253
Willow	143
Wine	117, 183, 187, 223, 231, 235
Wine of Antimony	123, 213, 215, 253
Wine of Spicae	213
Wintergreen	65, 103, 121, 127, 153, 253, 275, 287
Witch Hazel Sumac	35
Wormseed	181
Wormwood	61, 141, 143, 175, 179, 181, 225, 271, 287
Yarrow	143
Yeast	51, 61, 69, 105, 273
Yellow Dock	151, 155, 199, 205, 247, 251, 255, 259
Yellow Jessamine	165
Yellow Ochre	111
Yellow Perilla	239

Yellow Wax	173, 219
Zinc Acetate	127
Zinc Sulfate	167

Index of Diseases

Ague (malaria)	47, 57, 63, 109, 135, 143, 163, 201, 237, 239, 263, 271, 275
Amenorrhea	207
Asthma	137, 201, 209, 267, 289
Bathing	121, 173
Bed Ticks	97
Bellyache in Horses	59
Bleeding of the Lungs	167
Blood	251, 255, 285
Bots in Horses	59
Bone Pain	137
Bowel Disease	69, 201
Bronchitis	267
Broken Breast	201, 203
Bruise	41, 109, 145, 175, 199, 201, 207, 217, 253
Burns	63, 109, 201
Callus	41
Cancer	129, 155, 191, 197, 199
Canker	35, 201, 237
Captive Habits	289
Causativeness	39, 209
Chaps	227
Chilblains	109, 113, 191, 201, 203, 271, 283
Cholera	143, 189, 201, 203, 217, 223, 269, 289
Cholera Morbus	131, 193, 201, 217, 269
Clap	51, 65, 277, 281
Cold	53, 109, 201, 287
Cold Head	227
Colic	131, 165, 233, 285
Contraction of Cords, Sinews	207, 223, 253

Constipation	269
Contusions	201
Convulsions	267
Corns	49, 143, 197, 219, 263
Cough	37, 45, 53, 115, 135, 137, 147, 161, 181, 183, 201, 207, 209, 213, 215, 229, 253
Cramps	109, 209
Croup	117, 119, 137, 267, 289
Cuts	63, 109, 119, 145, 233, 251, 279
Diarrhea	53, 69, 131, 149, 165, 193, 227, 261, 269
Diphtheria	131, 243
Dropsy	119, 137, 195, 209
Dysentery	41, 43, 163, 165, 227, 269
Dysmenorrhea	159
Dyspepsia	203, 209, 269, 289
Epilepsy	133
Eruption on the Face	169
Eye Matter	117, 125, 193
Eye Wash	183
Faintness	211
Faintness of the Stomach	209
Female Weakness	207, 223
Fever	159, 165, 201, 239, 275
Fever Sores	147, 167, 243, 279
Fistula's Corking	109, 263
Fits	137
Flatulence	181
Frozen Limbs	109
Fluor Albus	209, 239
Galling of the Saddle	243

Gangrene	109, 279
Glandular Swellings	205
Gleet	281
Goiter	191
Gonorrhea	65, 137, 165, 167, 177, 189, 209, 251, 257, 281
Gravel	57, 137, 209
Gripes	181
Hare Flesh	109
Hydrophobia	149, 219
Indigestion	39
Inflammation	207, 237, 253
Itch	55-59, 133, 279
Jaundice	39
Kidney	201
Leukorrhea	189, 207
Lip Salve	183
Liver	161, 165, 171, 201, 209, 241, 251, 259
Loss of Appetite	39, 209
Lumbago	271
Lumps	237
Lungs	141, 157, 251, 259
Mildew	111
Moles	197, 263
Morbid Growth on Beasts	263
Mosquitos	113
Moths	111
Nausea	165
Nervous Pains	109, 131, 137, 209, 223, 283
Neuralgia	109, 127, 129, 175, 221, 277
Old Sores	63, 109, 119, 145, 147, 251, 279

Pain in Back	109
Pain in Bowels	131, 155
Pain in Breast	137, 209, 271
Pain in Chest	55
Pain in Ear	253
Pain in Head	127, 201, 277
Pain in Joints	109, 271
Pain in Side	109, 271
Pain in Stomach	39, 131, 155
Painful Menstruation	159
Painter's colic	201
Palpebra Muscles	207, 253
Palpitation	211
Paraphimosis	283
Phthisic Piles	201
Phimosis	283
Piles	219, 227, 269
Pimples	123
Pleurisy	271
Poll Evil	109, 263
Psalt-Rhuma	147, 227
Pulmonary	49
Quinsy	231, 239, 271
Restless Children	181
Restoring the Hair	187
Rheumatism	61, 109, 131, 173, 175, 191, 201, 207, 223, 225, 249, 253, 271, 283, 289
Rickets	271
Ringworm	127, 197, 263
Saddle Gall	109
Scalds	63, 109, 207, 253
Scalp Head Morphea	233

Scenting	211
Sciatica	109, 289
Scrofula	147, 201, 205, 207, 253, 255
Scrofulous Sores	119, 191, 199
Sore Eyes	45, 207
Sore Legs	109
Sore Throat	239
Sores	227, 251
Sour Stomach	181
Spasm	131, 191, 271
Spasmodic Attacks	157, 289
Spleen	231
Sprain	41, 109, 175, 199, 201, 207, 253, 283
Stiffness of the Joints	41, 191, 199, 283
Stifle	109
Stomach	121
Strains	175, 217
Sweeney	109
Swelled Neck	191
Swelled Testicle	281
Swelling	41, 191, 217, 271, 283
Syphilis	255
Tape Worm	179
Tetters	197, 227, 263
Tic Douloureux	109, 271
Tight Erections	283
Tightness of the Breast	239
Tightness of the Sinews	41
Tinea Capitis	233
Toothache	109, 127, 175, 201, 263, 271
Tumors	155, 191, 205
Ulcers	109, 167, 239, 179

Venereal	51
Vomiting	165
Warts	197, 263
Weak Stomach	55, 147, 201
Weakness of the Back	207
White Swellings	203, 271, 283
Whooping Cough	267
Wind Colic	181
Wind Gall	109, 263
Worms	43, 135, 139, 175, 181, 287
Wounds	109, 119, 207, 233, 253, 279

Food, other Recipes, Miscellaneous

Adhesive Plaster	63, 115
Antiphlogistic	237
Bathing Drops	121, 173
Birds Nest Pudding	91
Black Ink	273
Brandy Red	115
Bread	93
Carbonated Beer	69
Case Harden	237
Cement for Cisterns	229
Cider	101
Cider Cake	91
Cologne	179, 231
Colours	111
Common Loaf Cake	83
Cookies	75, 77, 85, 93
Cooling Plaster	237
Corn Meal Cakes	73
Costive Habits	285
Cream Cake	87
Cream Nectar	103
Crockers	81
Currant Wine	287
Custard	95
Elderberry Wine	273
Emmenagogue	65, 195
Emory for Inside of Barrels	237
Films	183
French Loaf	93
Fruit Cake	81
Genuine Whigs	75

Ginger Beer	69
Ginger Bread	81, 91, 93
Grease Spots	99
Green	89
Hams	111
Harrison Cake	85
Hiera Picra	53
How to Cut an Acquaintance	115
Housel's Washing Solution	130
Hungary Water	211
Ice Cream	71-73
Icing for Cake	83
Imitation Oysters	95
Indelible Ink	87
Japan Liquid Blacking	101
Jumbles	75
Kings Cake	87
Lavendar Water	211
Little Cake	79
Mead	103
Measure Cake	79
Medicated Indian Oil	107
Mildew	109
Mother's Relief	289
Muffins	77
Number Cake	77
Nut Cake	77
Paint	111
Perfume Clothes	111
Pill Coating	289
Plaster	217, 279, 285, 287
Plum Cake	79

Pound Cake	87, 89
Pudding	89
Puff Paste	81
Root Beer	59
Rusks	77
Soiled Coat	97
Sponge Cake	79
Spruce Beer	51, 55
Staining Guns	117, 235
Sunderland Pudding	87
The Real John Bull Pudding	85
To Clean Gloves	95
To Color Green	89
Vegetable Drops	263
Vegetable Powder	35
Vinegar	103
Wafers	75
Water Proof for Leather	113
Whip Syllabub	83
York Biscuit	81

www.ingramcontent.com/pod-product-compliance
Lightning Source LLC
Chambersburg PA
CBHW051801100526
44592CB00016B/2524